DEMENTIA *Arts*

To Charlotte
In poetry
xox
Gary Glynn

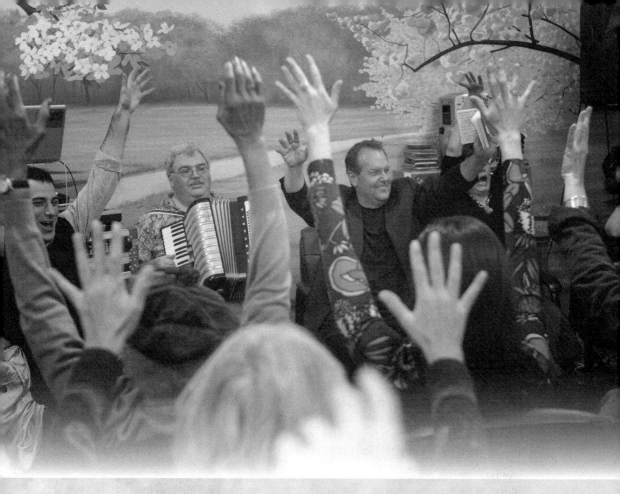

DEMENTIA *Arts*

Celebrating Creativity in Elder Care

Gary Glazner

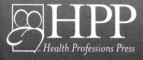

HPP
Health Professions Press

Baltimore • London • Sydney

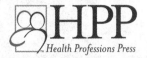

Health Professions Press, Inc.
Post Office Box 10624
Baltimore, Maryland 21285-0624

www.healthpropress.com

Interior and cover designs and typesetting by Mindy Dunn.
Manufactured in the United States of America by Versa Press, East Peoria, Illinois.

Every effort has been made to trace the ownership of all copyrighted material and to secure the necessary permission to reprint these selections. In the event of any question arising as to the use of any material, the author and the publisher, while expressing regret for any inadvertent error, will be happy to make the necessary correction in future printings.

The publisher and the author cannot be held responsible for injury, mishap, or damages incurred during the use of or because of the activities in this book. The author recommends appropriate and reasonable consideration be given based on the capability of each participant.

The individuals described in this book are real people whose situations are based on the author's experiences. In most instances, names and identifying details have been changed to protect confidentiality. Any real names and identifying details are used with permission.

All unpublished poetry is used with permission and remains the copyright of the poem's author or authors. All poems by Gary Glazner remain copyrighted to Gary Glazner. All other poetry is used with permission or is public domain.

All photographs, except for the Glazner family photographs, were taken by Michael Hagedorn and are used with permission. The Glazner family photographs are provided courtesy of the Glazner Family Trust.

Library of Congress Cataloging-in-Publication Data

Glazner, Gary, 1957– author.
  Dementia arts : celebrating creativity in elder care / by Gary Glazner.
    p. ; cm.
  Includes bibliographical references and index.
  ISBN 978-1-938870-11-8 (paper)
  I. Title.
  [DNLM: 1. Dementia—therapy. 2. Caregivers—psychology. 3. Creativity. 4. Dementia—psychology. 5. Poetry as Topic. 6. Sensory Art Therapies. WT 155]
  RC455.4.A77   616.89'1656—dc23   2014017897

British Library Cataloguing in Publication data are available from the British Library.

E-book edition: ISBN 978-1-938870-31-6

Contents

Recipes for Engagement

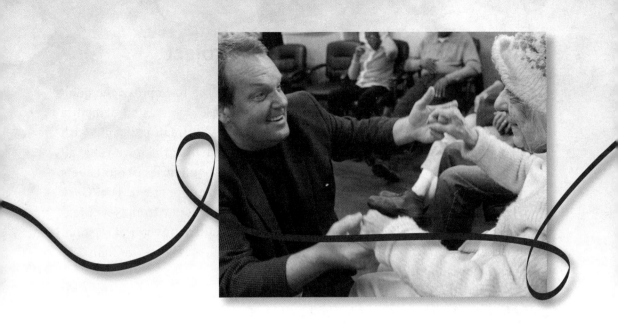

About the Author

Gary Glazner is the founder and Executive Director of the Alzheimer's Poetry Project (APP). Under Glazner's leadership, the APP received the 2013 Rosalinde Gilbert Innovations in Alzheimer's Disease Caregiving Legacy Award and the 2012 MetLife Foundation Creativity and Aging in America Leadership Award in the category of Community Engagement. The National Endowment for the Arts listed the APP as a "best practice" for their Arts and Aging initiative.

Glazner is an internationally recognized speaker and expert on using poetry with people living with Alzheimer's disease and related dementia and has given talks at more than 30 conferences for groups including the Alzheimer's Association; Alzheimer's Foundation of America; Global Alliance for Arts and Health; Grant Makers in the Arts; Institut für Bildung und Kultur; Korean Arts and Culture Education Service; Pioneer Network; and the U.S. Veterans Administration.

NBC's *Today* show, *PBS NewsHour*, NPR's *All Things Considered*, and Voice of America have featured segments on Glazner's work. HarperCollins, W.W. Norton, and Salon.com have published his work. Glazner has worked with many institutions using their art to inspire the performance and creation of poetry by people living with memory loss, including the Brooklyn Museum, Museum of Modern Art, Minneapolis Institute of Art, Orlando Art Museum, Neuberger Museum of Art, New Mexico History Museum, SPARK! Alliance (of museums in Wisconsin and Minnesota), and Toledo Art Museum.

About the Alzheimer's Poetry Project

The goal of the **Alzheimer's Poetry Project (APP)** is to improve the quality of life of people living with Alzheimer's disease and related dementia by facilitating creative expression through poetry. By treating people with dementia with dignity and by valuing them, we are telling them we value all members of our community. Further, we do not set boundaries in our beliefs in what is possible for people with memory impairment to create. Poet Gary Glazner founded the APP in 2003 with $300 in seed money from New Mexico Literary Arts. The APP is facilitated by an executive director, 3 regional directors, 17 project artists, and 10 volunteers and averages more than 200 poetry workshops each year.

In 2010, the U.S. Embassy in Berlin funded a pilot project for the APP in Germany. This work led to the funding of a pilot project for the APP in Poland in 2012 by the U.S. Embassy in Warsaw. Also in 2012, Glazner led a workshop on using poetry with people living with dementia at the Korean Arts and Culture Education Service International Arts Education Conference in Seoul. In 2013, Glazner was invited to start the APP in Australia as part of the 5th Annual The Art of Good Health and Wellbeing International Arts and Health Conference. Glazner was part of a delegation that met with the Minister of Aging for New South Wales to develop policy on arts in aging.

In 2012, the APP produced Dementia Arts on Capitol Hill (DACH), a week-long exhibit in the Rotunda of the Senate Office Building, with the support of the offices of Senators Edward Markey (MA), lead author of the National Alzheimer's Project Act (Public Law 111-375), and Tom Udall (NM). DACH included a panel briefing on dementia arts research. As a direct result of the panel, the APP received funding from the Alzheimer's Foundation of America for a pilot project to study dementia arts in 2014. Named the Dementia Arts Research Ensemble (DARE), participants include Kate de Medeiros, Ph.D., Assistant Professor of Gerontology and Scripps Fellow, Miami University; Jennifer M. Kinney, Ph.D., Professor, Department of Sociology & Gerontology, Scripps Research Fellow, and Affiliate, Department of Psychology; and Daniel Kaplan, Ph.D., Columbia University School of Social Work and postdoctoral research fellow at the Institute for Geriatric Psychiatry at Weill Cornell Medical College. Also participating in DARE are Anne Basting, TimeSlips; Maria Genné, KAIROS Dance; and Judith Kate Friedman, Songwriting Works.

The APP is unique in its cross-cultural reach in having provided programming in German, Hebrew, Hmong, Korean, Mandarin, Polish, and Spanish. Since 2004, the APP has taught techniques to more than 3,000 care partners and healthcare professionals through conference workshops and staff training. To date, the APP has held programming in 24 states and internationally in Australia, Germany, Poland, and South Korea, serving more than 20,000 people living with dementia. (Contact the APP at http://www.alzpoetry.com)

About the Institute of Dementia Arts and Education

In 2014, poet Gary Glazner founded the **Institute of Dementia Arts and Education (IDEA)** as a new initiative to use innovative nonpharmacological arts interventions to improve the quality of life of people living with memory loss as well as the health of their care partners and families. IDEA provides training and tools to teach creative aging methods to artists, family members, healthcare workers, teachers, and students of all ages. IDEA facilitates the training through shared models of best practices. IDEA's mission is to open our minds and hearts to the creativity of people navigating memory loss. We challenge ourselves to explore and create as well as to advance our knowledge of how to best serve each person living with dementia and his or her family—today. (Contact IDEA at http://www.dementiaarts.com)

Acknowledgments

To the people and families navigating memory loss, deep thanks for allowing me into your lives. It is an honor to serve you.

To Margaret Victor, my darling wife, a bouquet of thanks for your love and support and for being my first reader.

To my brothers, Kevin and Lon Glazner, and their families, thanks for your support and humor.

To Michael Hagedorn, photographer extraordinaire, thanks for your friendship, talent, and the generous use of your photographs. This book is better for your eye and skill at capturing the moment.

To Carol Steinberg and the Alzheimer's Foundation of America, thanks for giving me my first conference-speaking engagement and for all the years of support.

To Margery Pabst and the Pabst Charitable Foundation for the Arts, thanks for your years of support and for your guidance in deepening the work.

To Steve Young and the Poetry Foundation, thanks for your vision, your years of support, and your constant advocacy for poetry.

To Helen Ramon and the Helen Bader Foundation, thanks for your years of support and for teaching me about Friday fish fries in Wisconsin.

To Gay Hannah and the board and staff of the National Center for Creative Aging, thanks for your leadership and tireless work in developing the creative aging field.

To Christopher Nadeau and Josephine Brown of New York Memory Center, thanks for your support and giving me a home base.

To Jennie Smith-Peers and Elders Share the Arts, thanks for your inspiration and for challenging me to never stop growing as an artist.

To John and Susan McFadden, thanks for your friendship, delicious drinks and dinners, and leadership in creating dementia-friendly communities.

To Tom Leech, Director of the Press at the Palace of the Governors, thanks for your partnership at the New Mexico History Museum, as well as for your friendship, support, and opening my eyes to fine printing and old presses.

To Jane and Gary Tygesson, thanks for your partnership at the Minneapolis Institute of Arts, the amazing food, and a home away from home.

To Francesca Rosenberg, thanks for your partnership at the Museum of Modern Art and for fulfilling my dream to stand close to Van Gogh's *Starry Night* and recite poetry.

To Julie Chávez and Cecilia González and everyone at Health Professions Press, thanks for all your hard work and support in shaping the book.

To all the poets who have worked with the Alzheimer's Poetry Project through the years, I offer my unending gratitude. In no particular order and apologies in advance for those I have not included: Christopher Lane (1972–2012); Lars Rupple; Wolf Hogekamp; Zoë Bird; Rachel Moritz; Michelle Otero; Valerie Martínez; Joanne Dwyer; Beth Lisick; Lisa Marie Brodsky Auter; Fabu Carter; Don McIver; Marc Smith; Robbie Telfer; Mary Fons; Cari Griffo; Bohdan Piasecki; Natalia Malek; Weronika Lewandowska; Wojciech Cicho; Grzegorz Bruszewski; Jan Kowalewicz; Henrikje Stanze; Pauline Füg; Fabian "Farbeon" Saucedo; and DJ Rabbi-Darkside and the Purple Cow Poets.

To all the artists dedicated to serving people living with memory loss, thanks for including me in the community.

To all the poets, living and dead, whose work we have used in the Alzheimer's Poetry Project, it is an honor to give breath to your work and bring your poems to life each day.

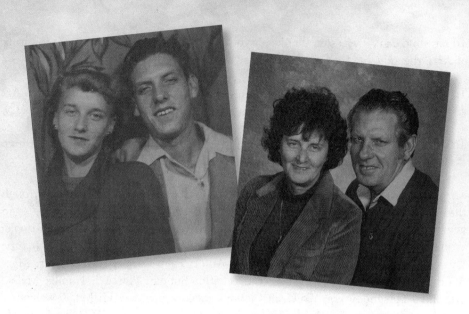

*This book is dedicated in loving memory to Frankie and Billy Glazner
and to all the people I have had the honor of working with.*

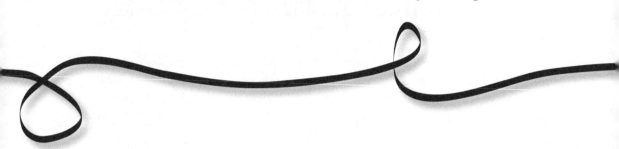

My mind's not at all a blank slate,
Though I cannot keep track of the date
    Or the day of the week,
    And facts play hide-and-seek,
For my mind to be blank would be great.

Instead it is wired like spaghetti;
It conflates the important and petty;
    The connections of things
    Are like tangles of strings
Or like celebratory confetti.

STUART HALL

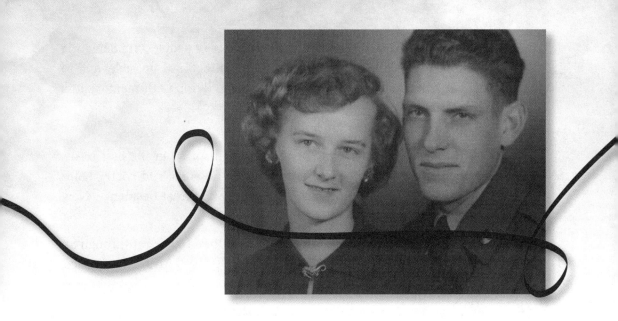

Introduction

In 1980, when I first began to write and study poetry, I had a job delivering flowers and one of the places I delivered to was a convalescent home. Walking the florescent lit, linoleum halls of the convalescent home, I could hear people crying out from their beds. The smell of bleach covering urine and the solitary wail of those voices are still vivid after more than 30 years.

At the core of my work with the Alzheimer's Poetry Project (APP) is the desire to respond to those voices.

It is often said that the person in the late-stage of dementia lives in the moment. Short-term memory has faded and as the disease continues to progress, he or she remembers less and less from the past. On many occasions a person with dementia I have laughed, played, and recited poems with, when I am saying good-bye, will ask,

Who are you?

I'm Gary.

What do you do?

I am a poet.

Will you do poetry with us?

Memories of the laughs and the time spent playing together and the poems shared have gone from their minds. This moment, right this instant, is the person's reality.

This book has a dual purpose: to make the lives of people with dementia and that moment of connection as rich and meaningful as possible, and to challenge our belief in what is possible for people living with memory loss to create.

What have people with dementia told us?

- "To me, and I think to many people, poetry brings out the best in us. For people like us with Alzheimer's, we get nervous, and poetry helps calm us. You ask us to do things." (Martha, 80th Street Residence, New York, NY)

- "I have lived here a year and this is the first time I have sat through an activity to the end. You made us all poets." (Jean, Attic Angel Place, Madison, WI)

- "My name is Jim. I am a person with Alzheimer's. We attended the session this evening where we did an interactive development of a song. It was very engaging. It brought us out of our shells. It helps both those caregivers who are, quote, 'normal' and those of us with the disease to have fun. That gets to the gist of improving the quality of life of those with Alzheimer's. We're not just looking for a cure here. We're looking for an improved lifestyle, and this helped." (Jim, participant in Dementia Arts on Capitol Hill, Washington, D.C.)

These responses to APP's work are representative of the dementia community as a whole. What do we learn from them?

- Martha liked being asked to do things, as opposed to the many times people did not even bother to see what she was capable of doing.

- Jean was amazed at how engaged she was by poetry and happily surprised to find that she could be a poet.

- Jim voices the frustration of so many people in dementia community that while, yes, we all want a cure, as a society we also desperately need to figure out what we can do now, today, at this moment.

Our belief in the creativity of people living with memory loss strengthens us as a community in connecting us to them as human beings. The goal of this book is to provide compelling examples to the question of what can be done today to improve the quality of life of people living with dementia and their families. My hope is to help caregivers, interested community members, and other artists such as myself have the strength and heart to answer that call.

WE ARE FORGET
GARY GLAZNER

We are the words we have forgotten.
We are shifting and pacing.
We wrote this poem.
It's a pretty poem.
Can you bake a cherry pie?
Never more, never more.
We have no horizon.
We don't recall washing or eating
or what you just said.
Ask me my name.
Ask me if I have children.
You are my daughter?
Give me a kiss, brush my hair,
put me to bed clean,
hold me as I fall asleep.
Light washing over us moment, moment.
Our handwriting is beautiful
twists and loops of letters.
We can't remember our hands.
Our ears are wishful
we can't remember our ears.
We can speak every language,
we can't remember our mouths.
We are porous.
We are the past.
We are forget.

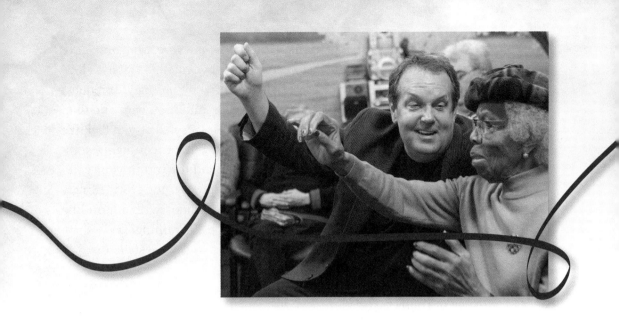

Ways to Use This Book

While my work with the Alzheimer's Poetry Project (APP) focuses on people living with memory loss, many of the techniques can be used with any elders and many of the lessons may also be adapted to include children.

Each of the chapters begins with a story on using creativity. In addition to writing about my experience with poetry, I offer examples of how to combine poetry with dance, improvisation, music, and visual art.

Many of the chapters end with a "recipe" for creativity, an activity that offers a lesson in communication and interaction built around art. One reason I use a recipe format is that I want engaging in the arts to feel familiar. By placing the art instruction in a format many people use on a daily basis, I hope it will create a playful experience and break down any concerns one may have about lack of creativity. I also hope to connect the idea of using art and humor as nourishment and incorporate the celebratory feeling of coming together to share a meal. Some of the recipes will be playful and others more like a poem than instructional.

The book is also an opportunity to introduce you to many of the wonderful people I have met while working in this field. The poet Craig Arnold once told me he thought of a successful poem as being like a fun dinner party. With that spirit, I invite you to join us at the table.

Please use this book daily like a cookbook. Come back to it again and again for sustenance. Your task is to bring its words and lessons to life by engaging people with dementia. I hope it is of use in your life as well as in the lives of those for whom you care.

As I began to envision how to shape this book, my wife, Margaret, gave me a gift of *The Essential New York Times Cookbook*, by Amanda Hesser. I love the author's helpful tone and was especially inspired by her playful request that using a certain technique would ruin the recipe, and "you won't do that, right? Because I'll lose sleep if you do. So don't!" Hesser makes you feel like you have a friend in the kitchen helping you out with encouraging comments, a cheerleader for food. I want to be that friend for you in your caregiving by being a cheerleader for art, dance, music, poetry, and storytelling.

You may wish to supplement the activities in this book with our on-line training (visit http://www.alzpoetry.com/On-Line%20Training/).

There are two chapters that step outside the story/recipe structure:

- Through the Looking Glass

- Biology of Poetry

Through the Looking Glass is my account of living in a skilled nursing facility for a week to help build empathy and better understand the lives of the people we serve doing this work.

Biology of Poetry pulls together various scientific studies and an essay on poetry as a memory tool. It uses the structure of a science fair hypothesis ("If [I do this], then [this will happen].") instead of a recipe to inform my understanding of why poetry evokes such a strong response from people living with memory loss and will hopefully serve as a blueprint for a research project.

This book seeks to entertain, inspire, guide, and help you in your journey as a caregiver, healthcare professional, teaching artist, friend or loved one, student or teacher, who in some way has been moved to want to help an elder have a better life.

How many more exercises such as this can you think of? Here is a secret; all poets and artists carry a notebook, because you never know when inspiration is going to strike. Be sure to keep a notebook with you to write your thoughts and perhaps your own recipes to help with care situations. You may also share them with us on the Alzheimer's Poetry Project blog.

I look forward to hearing from you. Or as they say, operators are standing by.

Please do not hesitate to reach out to me for help, comments, or just to say hello. You may contact me at garyglaznerpoet@gmail.com.

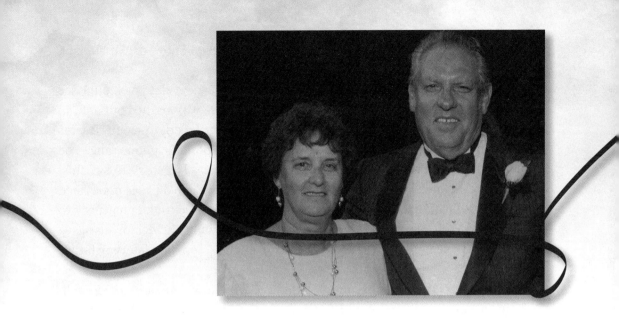

On Being a Caregiver

One of the reasons I am so driven to share poetry with people living with dementia is my own experience of being a caregiver. While my father did not have dementia, I was honored to be able to recite poems to him during his last days.

Listening may be the most important tool you possess as a caregiver. You listen and respond to your loved one. My first sign that something was wrong with my father was as I listened to his voice on the phone. We were heading home for Christmas and I had called to check in, confirm arrival times, and really to just say hello. His voice sounded so tired.

When we would say good-bye, being men we did not naturally say "I love you," but I had started telling my 82-year-old dad that I loved him. My aunt, Ann, had told me that my dad got a big kick out of it and even though it was hard for him, he said he loved me too and had shared with her, "Gary has started saying he loves me at the end of our phone calls, and now I listen for it and it is the best part of the call."

When I got off the phone, I told my wife, "He sounded so tired. I'm so glad we're going home for Christmas." Margaret and I had planned to visit her family first in southern California for Christmas Eve then fly north to be with my family on Christmas Day. I really wanted to hear my dad's voice again and I was worried about our last conversation, so I called him back. This time he told me, "I just feel so tired." I told Margaret, "I think we should change our plans and fly up right away." She calmed me down and we had a lovely Christmas Eve at her parent's home. It even snowed. We all sang "White Christmas" in our best Bing Crosby voices.

When we walked into my father's house the next day, we could see something was not right. It was as if some part of life was leached out of him. He was pale and frail and walking slow. He told us, "I went to see my doctor today and he should call with the results tonight." Soon, the phone rang. The doctor told my father that what he feared was true: "I'm sorry to say this, Bill, but you have liver cancer and there is nothing we can do." He prescribed a pain medication and my brother and I offered to drive to the pharmacy to pick it up. When we got in the car, my brother said, "The doctor just gave him a death sentence." We sat for a while in silence. Ten days later my father was dead.

I tell you this story because I want to let you know you are not alone in being a caregiver. You do not have to make the journey alone. I learned a lot about listening to my father, the doctors and nurses, and my brothers. The hospice that cared for him was all about listening and encouraged me to slow down, listen to my thoughts, and write them down as a way of helping me take care of myself during this difficult time.

In going through our father's papers, I found a note he had written about growing up in Oklahoma:

> My earliest memories are of our farm in Blair. We lived in a two-room house. The "bathroom" consisted of a one-hole outhouse and, for Saturday nights, a large washtub. There were no kids living close by, so I mostly played alone. My game of choice was pretending the tumbleweeds were cattle and I would chase them on a stick horse and rope them with a heavy cord. I would then drag them back to the barn and put them in the corral. With the Oklahoma wind always blowing this was quite a job.

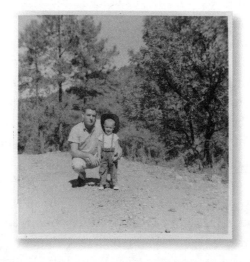

Please allow me to share a poem I wrote about being a caregiver for my father, Billy, at the end of his life:

THE I.V. WALTZ
GARY GLAZNER
(AFTER THEODORE ROETHKE)

The morphine on your breath
Could make a grown man dizzy.

His hands on my shoulders,
he helps to lift himself up.
I.V. stand, maypole ribbons
of tube and power cord.
We step, step, stop,
step, step, steady,
our way to the toilet,
rolling the stand after us.
He can sit up on his own,
I give him a moment.
Snap on surgical gloves,
gently clean him.
Reverse our papa waltz,
lay him down to rest.

Trying to look busy,
listening for his death.

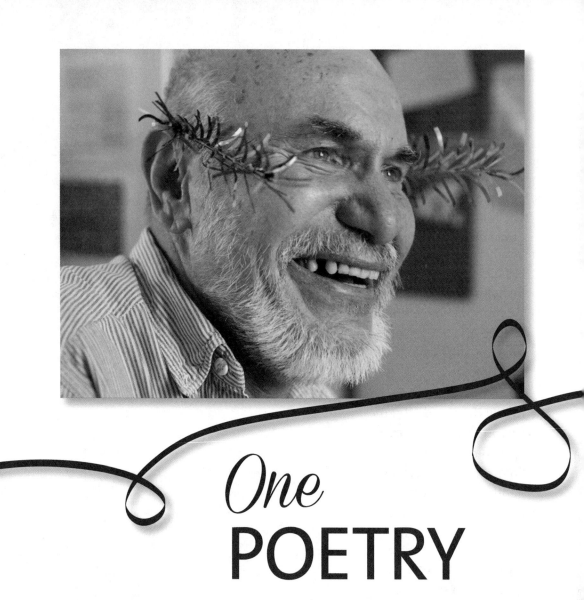

One
POETRY

On Starting the Alzheimer's Poetry Project and Sharing Poems with a Loved One

In 1997, seventeen years after my first experience delivering flowers in the nursing home, I desperately wanted to quit working at the flower shop and become a full-time poet. As a way to help incorporate more poetry into my life, I applied for a grant to use poetry at one of three local facilities: two were convalescent homes and one was an adult day care center for people living with Alzheimer's disease.

I was awarded the grant to conduct a poetry workshop at the adult day care center. There was no additional instruction, just simply "use poetry." My initial moment of inspiration was after observing a man with his head down, not participating, and seemingly unaware of his surroundings. I chose to share the Longfellow poem, "The Arrow and the Song." Upon reciting, "I shot an arrow into the air," the man's eyes popped open and he responded, "It fell to earth, I knew not where." Suddenly, he was able to participate. This moment showed me how useful poetry could be in engaging this community. I was and remain inspired to make my life's work serving people who are living with dementia, which led me to found the Alzheimer's Poetry Project (APP).

During that same time, my mother, Frankie, had terminal cancer. Brain tumors and morphine were causing dementia-like behavior. Billy, my father, called to say she was agitated and asking for cherry ice cream. As I arrived at their house and reached into the back seat of the car, sitting next to the bag with the ice cream were all of the poetry books from the workshop. In a flash, I saw myself reading the poems to my mother.

My parents were childhood sweethearts from the young ages of 5 and 6. My mother had teased my dad with, "Can she bake a cherry pie, Billy boy, Billy boy." We all recited the words. It was strikingly clear to me that poetry could be of use to people with dementia. During the time leading up to her death about a month later, I was able to continue to share poetry with her.

Outside their bedroom window, my father had hung a hummingbird feeder. From her deathbed my mother could watch the birds flutter and sip the red sugar water. Beyond the feeder was their garden. The garden was mostly flowers, yellow cymbidium orchids and orange dahlias with blooms as big as your head. My mother and father loved picking oranges from their orange tree. Perhaps the most magical bit of nature for people having grown up in dust bowl Oklahoma was fresh orange juice from a tree they had planted.

Growing up, their garden always had rows of tomato plants. My toddler brother, Kevin, would sink his teeth into ripe fruit, but leave them hanging on the vine. When you went to pick the tomatoes, each one had little rows of tiny bite marks. Chomp, grin, chomp, grin, chomp, grin, Kevin!

The poem that had the most resonance for me to share with my mother was Shakespeare's Sonnet 18 with its gorgeous opening lines:

Shall I compare thee to a summer's day?
Thou art more lovely and more temperate:
Rough winds do shake the darling buds of May,

As my mother was born in May and her hospice was taking place in May, that third line had particular significance. I would quietly read the poem to her and would often repeat the closing lines, among the most famous in the English language:

So long as men can breathe or eyes can see,
So long lives this and this gives life to thee.

These closing lines echoed what I wanted to say to my mother—that in the face of hopefulness, love expressed through poetry can make the love live forever. I often use Sonnet 18 in my work with the APP.

How to Select a Poem

For selecting poems to use with my mother, I had a stack of books with me. It is doubtful you will be lugging around a small library, so as an alternative you can use any Internet search engine (Google, Yahoo, Internet Explorer, etc.) to easily find a poem of almost any theme that might be of interest to your loved one. A trip to the library to browse the poetry stacks can also be fruitful and relaxing. Lastly, feel free to email me at gary@alzpoetry.com and I will be happy to find the perfect poem for your loved one.

Sample poetry themes include the following:

- flowers, gardens, the outdoors
- colors
- seasons (spring, summer, autumn, winter)
- children
- weather (sunshine, snow, rain, fog)
- food
- sports (fishing, baseball, football)
- animals

The following websites have built in search engines to find poems by theme or by poet:

Poetry Foundation (http://www.poetryfoundation.org)

Academy of American Poets (http://www.poets.org)

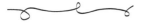

THE POEM REMEMBERS *(excerpt)*
MICHELLE OTERO
(for the Alzheimer's Poetry Project)

The poem remembers when yesterday was yesterday.
Today is today.
In this moment, it is all the same.
We are all the same. We are the poem.
We remember.

MY MOTHER'S SUMMER POEM

INGREDIENTS:

1 poem
1 mother
1 son

SERVES 2

INSTRUCTIONS:

1. Read the poem with humor and playfulness.

2. Read the poem with quiet reflection.

3. Play with repeating lines that have a particular significance.

SONNET 18
WILLIAM SHAKESPEARE

Shall I compare thee to a summer's day?
Thou art more lovely and more temperate:
Rough winds do shake the darling buds of May,
And summer's lease hath all too short a date:
Sometime too hot the eye of heaven shines,
And often is his gold complexion dimm'd;
And every fair from fair sometime declines,
By chance or nature's changing course untrimm'd;
But thy eternal summer shall not fade
Nor lose possession of that fair thou owest;
Nor shall Death brag thou wander'st in his shade,
When in eternal lines to time thou growest:
So long as men can breathe or eyes can see,
So long lives this and this gives life to thee.

Basic Principles of the Alzheimer's Poetry Project, with a Sprinkling of Poetry Tips

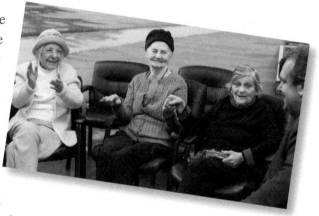

The principles or techniques of the Alzheimer's Poetry Project may be combined in myriad ways. They are like the basic ingredients to a favorite recipe. How you combine them, the amount of time you allot to each, and the order in which you do them will all be a part of the decision making process you will engage in when working with your loved one or activity participant.

The chapters that follow delve into each of the techniques in more depth, including looking at ways to combine them with dance, exercise, music, storytelling, and visual art. They also include suggestions for working with participants of all ages. (You can also see examples of these techniques at APP's YouTube Channel: http://www.youtube.com/user/alzpoetry)

Tips for Building a Poetry Session

The following tips define the structure of a poetry session and offer some common sense methods that I have found particularly useful in working with people living with memory loss. The sessions that APP conducts take place in assisted living, adult day care, and senior centers. You may also use these techniques to perform and create poems one-on-one in a home setting with your loved one.

Group Size: The size of the group will vary depending on the needs of the facility. Our groups have ranged in size from one person to up to 85 people. An average size group for APP would be in the 10-to-15-person range. While APP techniques and methods may work with any size group, for larger groups the poetry session becomes more of a performance in order to hold the participants' attention. For at-home programming, the tone is more conversational and normally takes less time than for a group session.

Poem Selection: Select a group of poems. They may be linked by theme (e.g., spring).

Length of Session: The typical length of a poetry session would be an hour. The session can be divided into 30 minutes of performing poems and 30 minutes of creating a new poem. Each session ends with the performance of a new work.

Seating Arrangement: If possible, have everyone sit in a circle.

Getting Started: First, greet everyone. Start by shaking everyone's hand and saying hello. Listen to how each person responds and interacts with you. Can the person hear you? If you say your name, does the person say his or her name? This quick check in will help you work together. It gives you a sense of each participant's ability to respond to social cues. Tell the group that you will be performing and creating poems with them.

- While you may be seated during the session, you may also move closer to the participants and kneel so you are not always standing over them when talking.

- You may also choose to stand and recite a poem to give it emphasis.

Encouraging Participation: Reinforce a participant's comments or responses by repeating them and giving praise for what each person says. Listen for when someone uses humor or creativity and repeat what the person said to be sure the group heard it and can respond. This is especially effective with people living with memory loss, as it gives a second chance to hear a joke or comment.

- Ask permission before asking a question: "May I ask you a question, please?"

Ending the Session: At the end of the session, thank the participants for their creativity and performance.

Main Techniques Used to Build a Poetry Session

Once you have structured the poetry session, use the following techniques to engage the participants.

Engage the Group in Call and Response

Recite a line of high-energy poetry. Have the group echo you. This is an aerobic activity that helps to build and hold attention. Begin by saying a few lines or even just a word. You are getting the group warmed up. After you say a line, let the group respond. Refrain from repeating the line with them; this will help give space for their voices. If you are reciting just a few lines from a longer poem, once you end the call and response ask the group if they want to hear the whole poem and, if so, with feeling recite it for them or a longer section of the poem.

Use Poems as Discussion Starters

Use poems as a flash point for discussions. Build questions based on the subject matter of the poem. Reinforce the responses by reciting lines from the poem using the technique of call and response.

Incorporate Props

Use items the group can smell, feel, and hold. Build a program around the props. Examples of props include leaves and branches for a tree- or nature-themed poem, a bouquet of flowers for a floral-themed poem, and a balloon or beach ball to play catch with for a sports-themed poem.

Create a Group Poem

Use the simple prompt of asking an open-ended question to begin creating a group poem. Choose a classic poem as the model and then base the prompt on the subject matter of the poem (e.g., "Daffodils" by Wordsworth). Ask what spring smells, tastes, sounds, looks, and feels like. Write down the participants' responses as the lines of the poem.

Call and Response

The core concept of the Alzheimer's Poetry Project is call and response, when the session leader recites a line of poetry and then has the group echo back the words. It is a technique I have used in working with everyone from preschool children to 100-year old elders. I have used it with large groups and one-on-one in the home. A majority of the lessons in this book include an element of call and response.

My interest in multi-voice poetry performance grew from my work in the poetry slam grassroots movement. Marc Smith coined the term *poetry slam* and started the performance competition in Chicago in the late 1980s. In a poetry slam, it is common for the teams to work together and perform what are known as "group poems."

I think one of the reasons that call and response works so well is that it is embedded in our culture in many ways. You find call and response in music forms, especially gospel, blues, and jazz. Counterpoint in classical music can be a form of call and response. You also see call and response used in yoga classes, with the Kirtan, which was developed in India. *Kirtan* from Sanskrit means "to repeat." In the Occupy movement of 2011, we saw a creative use of call and response renamed the "human microphone." Call and response is also found in religious ceremonies throughout the world (e.g., the shouting out of "amen" in Baptist ceremonies; the intoning of catholic litanies). The reciting of wedding vows is perhaps the most famous example of call and response.

Call and response is an effective technique in reaching people living with dementia. Because participants are following along in unison, it allows for a high success rate for many elders, even for those in the late stage of dementia whose language skills are severely reduced.

Call and response uses what is known as "echoic memory" which is "a brief mental echo that is thought to last for upwards of about three or four seconds after an auditory stimulus has been heard" (http://psychology. wikia.com/wiki/Echoic_memory). Echoic memory is also defined as "the ability to recapture the exact impression of a sound shortly after the sound has finished" (http://www.thefreedictionary.com/echoic + memory).

The time span of four seconds is very close to the length of time it takes to say a line of poetry written in iambic pentameter (a line of verse consisting of five metrical feet). Many of our most loved and well-known poems use this rhythm and are perfectly suited for call and response.

Incorporating echoic memory sidesteps the need for the participant to access his or her short-term memory by encouraging the person to repeat a phrase just heard. Echoic memory seems to remain intact even in late-stage dementia.

A 2004 study showed that reciting poetry using the technique of call and response had an aerobic benefit and reduced stress indicators (http://ajpheart.physiology.org/content/287/2/H579). In the study researchers used call and response in combination with movement to regulate a subject's breathing: "The subject listened to the text recited by the therapist without lifting the arms (but continued walking) and subsequently repeated it in the therapist's fashion."

Anecdotally, when we at APP engage people in call and response, we see their affect brighten; they become more social, alert, and engaged. The artistic focus of using call and response is on participant creativity, inspired by energetic and associative performance.

The approach is simple: the session leader chooses several lines of poetry, either a short poem or an excerpt that can stand alone, and leads the group in reciting it. Lines should be about four seconds long. Sometimes it is helpful to break the line in half, as it gives the group fewer words to repeat back. Rhyming couplets work well, such as the ending of Sonnet 18 by William Shakespeare. The line breaks can be changed to read:

So long as men can breathe/
or eyes can see,/
So long lives this/
and this gives life to thee./

People respond eagerly to poems that are familiar or humorous, especially when the leader selects the most memorable lines. The following poems are among the ones that have received the strongest responses during APP sessions (a list of recommended poems is also available at www.alzpoetry/book.com):

"Tyger," by William Blake

"Rattlesnake Meat," by Ogden Nash

"I Wandered Lonely as a Cloud," by William Wordsworth

A key to being a successful session leader is the delivery of the lines of poetry. The leader needs to recite them loudly enough to be heard by everyone in the room, and they should be spoken at a speed that is not too fast to follow but that also maintains the poem's rhythm. It is important to articulate words well; this will be especially helpful for elders with hearing impairment. A smile and a lively energy will likely enliven participants as well.

The call and response technique can be effective with older adults with all levels of physical and cognitive abilities. Even those with late-stage memory impairment can successfully engage. For those who are losing language and are comfortable with touch, the session leader can kneel down before the person and recite the lines while moving the participant's hand to the rhythm. It is best first to orient the person to what is happening by saying something like, "I'm going to recite the poem and move your hand to the rhythm." Engaging an elder in this way often receives a positive response from the participant, who may start to move his or her lips, smile, or brighten in the eyes. You need to read the person's body language to see if he or she is open to being touched.

The technique can be used to perform original content that is created during a session as a way of unifying the group at closing. For example, it can be used to perform a story the group has created or comments the group has made about a piece of art they have observed during the session. Call and response also can be combined with movement or music activities. APP often uses the technique with the chair exercises that are common in assisted living and adult day care centers (chanting along with the movements). Also try using the technique in context with accomplishing daily activities, such as taking a shower or getting in and out of a car.

Be sure to find a partner to practice call and response with.

Using Poetry as a Discussion Starter

Purple Cow Hugs and
Warning Bad Pun Up Ahead

John was a retired lieutenant colonel. He had spent 30 years in the army and had an iron grip handshake. At the age of 90 he still crunched down on your hand like a vise. When I read a poem to John that he did not like, such as my rap version of "The Raven," he gave me the thumbs down. When I read a love poem he found sappy, like "How Do I Love Thee, Let Me Count the Ways," John played an imaginary violin.

I was reading love poems to a group at Sierra Vista Assisted Living Center in Santa Fe, New Mexico, on Valentine's Day, including "The Purple Cow," by Gelett Burgess:

I've never seen a purple cow
I hope I never see one
I can tell you anyhow
I'd rather see than be one.

Strangely, I do consider "The Purple Cow" a love poem. John was sitting with Rosy his wife of 55 years. I said "John, have you ever seen a purple cow?" He said, "No, but I married one." Now, that was a mean answer. Rosy gave him an elbow to his ribs. I knew then that their 55-year marriage was based on a shared sense of humor. At that moment a man in late-stage dementia had told a joke with perfect timing, and even Rosy had to laugh.

Poetry can be a very effective flash point for discussions. Using "The Purple Cow" as an example, I will ask if the person has ever seen a purple cow. Some common responses are "Only when I drink" or "Purple cow—

isn't that a cocktail?" The interaction builds energy and attention; you use the poem to pique the person's interest.

The idea is to step outside of our normal way of communicating by focusing the person on the lines of poetry and then asking questions about the imagery and themes of the poem. This type of participation may help an individual who is navigating memory loss to be present by drawing the person out and engaging him or her. By shifting back and forth between reciting the poem with the person using call and response and talking about the poem, you are helping him or her to focus. This can be a wonderful diversion from our regular patterns of conversation.

"The Purple Cow" was published in the San Francisco Chronicle. Burgess wrote a second verse:

I've never seen a purple cow
My eyes with tears are full.
I've never seen a purple cow
And I'm a purple bull.

Then the poem was published in newspapers all over the world and became so popular that people would often stop Burgess on the street and ask about it. So he wrote this retraction:

Confession: And a Portrait, Too, Upon a Background that I Rue!

Oh, yes, I wrote "The Purple Cow,"
I'm sorry now I wrote it!
But I can tell you anyhow,
I'll kill you if you quote it.

I was reciting the poem at St. Gabriel's Adult Day Center in Milwaukee, and one of the men said, "We are in a church. Can we do something about that last line?" So now I recite it as such:

Oh, yes, I wrote "The Purple Cow,"
I'm sorry now I wrote it!
But I can tell you anyhow,
I'll hug you if you quote it.

Then I give someone in the group a big hug.

Warning: Bad Pun Up Ahead

Often when using "The Purple Cow," I will lead the discussion into a horrible pun. It goes something like this:

Gary: What color milk do you think a purple cow would have?

Group: No matter what color the cow, the milk is always white. You don't get chocolate milk from a brown cow do you?

Gary: True, but imagine it was colored. What color might it be?

Group: Purple or lavender.

Gary: Okay, follow me on this, and I am warning you, there is a terrible pun up ahead.

You have a purple cow, it has purple milk: What is a juice or a drink we like that is purple?

Group: Grape juice.

Gary: Yes, now what happens to grape juice when it ages? When it ferments?

Group: It turns to wine.

Gary: Yes, okay, here we go. You have a purple cow, it has purple milk, it tastes like grape juice, it turns to wine. Is it *Cow-bernet?*

Group: AAAUUUUUUGGGGGHHHH!!

Once I was working in Baraboo, Wisconsin, and after engaging a group in this horrible pun a woman looked at me and said, "No, it's "Moooooooooo-erlot.""

GRANDMA'S GENTLY GUIDED GAB FEST

INGREDIENTS:

1 poem
2 (or more) curious minds

INSTRUCTIONS:

Use the poem as a discussion starter. Ask questions about the poem. For example, when I use "The Tyger," I ask if the group likes tigers. Often they say something like, "I wouldn't want to meet one in a dark alley."

Listen for funny or interesting comments and acknowledge what each person says. Perhaps even repeat what someone says (e.g., "Bob just said he likes tigers, but only in the zoo.")

We talk about if tigers are beautiful. What color are they? Would they be fun to ride? How do they compare to house cats? What are the similarities and the differences between the two?

Say, "I have a tiger by the _____." (Let them finish the sentence.)

"If he hollers, let him _____."

"I have a tiger in my _____."

This can work with any poem. After talking about the poem, reinforce the discussion by reciting the poem with the group using call and response.

Props

When I worked in the flower shop, it was easy for me to find props to bring to a poetry session to have the participants hold, smell, touch, or taste. But after my wife and I sold the business and I embarked on my life as a full-time poet, I was at a loss as to what to bring. We had moved to Santa Fe, New Mexico, and I was preparing for my first session at Sierra Vista Assisted Living Center. I was looking around and outside I saw the answer: snow!

I filled an ice chest full of snow. At the center I made snowballs and passed them around. The participants touched the snow. Many wanted to taste the snow and began to eat it. For some, the snow was too cold. At one point the activities director, Ruth Dennis, whispered, "Throw them at Gary."

Suddenly it was . . .

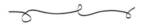

WHACK!

> Miles to go . . . SPLAT!

> Before I sleep . . . PLOP!

Snowballs are glistening
are you listening?
They are flying at me from every angle,
It's a beautiful sight
We're happy tonight

Fffffffmmmmmppp . . . Ouch!

It hit me that working

with this group was going

to be rewarding in ways

I had not expected.

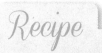

MS. JEN THOMPSON'S SPRING RAIN

INGREDIENTS:

1 misting spray bottle
1 basket of strawberries
1 punch bowl of fresh lemonade

INSTRUCTIONS:

Sing "April Showers" and "Raindrops Keep Falling on My Head" to the group. Lightly spray mist onto the participants' cheeks. Describe the feeling. Eat strawberries and drink lemonade. Talk about the taste, texture, and smell of the fruit and drink. Ask what spring evokes. Write down the responses, as these will become the lines of your poem. Perform the newly created poem.

This recipe was created by Jen Thompson.

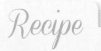
Recipe

BREWSTER VILLAGE'S FRIDAY FISH FRY

INGREDIENTS:

1 fishing pole with reel (put the hook in a cork)
1 tackle box (full of bobbers)
1 pair of thigh-high waders (optional)
1 creel full of fishing poems

FISHING POEM SUGGESTIONS:

"Fishing," by A. E. Stallings
"Cod," by Cheryl Savageau
"The Fish," by Elizabeth Bishop (Best to use an excerpt, as the poem is long. There are many beautiful passages.)

INSTRUCTIONS:

Fish out a few fishing poems. Pass around the rod and reel. Open the tackle box and pass around the bobbers. Talk about fishing. Tell a tall tale. Explore fishing through your senses. Expand the discussion to talk about lakes, swimming, or summer. How is fishing calming? Can being patient while fishing be applied to other aspects of life? Write down the participants' responses to form the lines of the poem. Perform the newly created poem.

This recipe was created by Carrie Platt, Megan Burns, and Evan Weiske.

Dr. London and Ocean
Creating a Poem Using Open-Ended Questions

Claudia, a caregiver, had called me on behalf of the wife of the man she was taking care of. The wife, Trudie, had attended a talk I had given the day before at the Napa Valley Alzheimer's Disease Education Conference hosted by the Northern California Chapter of the Alzheimer's Association. Trudie was wondering where she and her husband could get a copy of my poetry book. Claudia asked if I thought she could get it from a local bookstore. I told her I did not think that would be possible and asked where she was calling from. She said she was in San Rafael and was taking care of a man named Fred London, who was a retired doctor and who loved poetry. I told her I would be driving through San Rafael and I would love to come and work with her and Dr. London. I would also bring the book Dr. London and his wife were looking for: *Sparking Memories: The Alzheimer's Poetry Project Anthology.*

When I arrived, I told Dr. London I had heard he loved poetry and that I also loved poetry and wanted to share some poems with him. He was very polite, but said, "I have a tennis lesson today, and any other day would be fine, but not today." Claudia explained to him that they had changed the date of the tennis lesson. We then all sat down in the living room, where Claudia had stacked many of Dr. London's favorite poetry books.

I taught Claudia the technique of call and response. She and I recited "The Love Song of J. Alfred Prufrock," by T.S. Elliot; "Sonnet 18," by William Shakespeare; and "Anyone Lived in a Pretty How Town," by e.e. cummings. For fun we also recited "Rattlesnake Meat," by Ogden Nash. Dr. London and Claudia enjoyed saying the poems. We all laughed and had a fun time.

Dr. London had walked into the dining room, and I said to Claudia, "It looks like he is finished and we won't get a chance to create a poem together." He then came back into the room and asked if I knew the works of two poets: Allen Cohen and Constance Walker. I told him I did not know their work. (Later when I Googled them, I found that Cohen had founded the *San Fran-*

cisco Oracle, an underground newspaper. Walker is well known for her poem "Pray for Peace," which has been reprinted in more than twenty-five publications.) Dr. London then said, "If I don't write it down, it's shhhhhhh." I asked him if I could write down what he had just said and if we could try to create a poem together. He seemed pleased to agree and sat back down.

I asked Dr. London a series of questions to explore poetry through his senses, and using his responses we created this *ars poetica*, or "poem on the nature of poetry." I started by repeating his opening line, which had such a resonance regarding memory loss. That prompted him to look at the window and give a wonderful description of the rolling hills of Northern California.

Next I asked Dr. London what he thought of when he heard the word *poetry*, which led him to talk about Constance Walker and Robert Frost. I then asked him what a poem tasted like. This was, undoubtedly, a strange question, and so I encouraged him to use his imagination, as we do not normally think of poetry as having a taste.

After each question Dr. London would close his eyes, scrunching up his brow in concentration, and then the words would come pouring out so fast it was hard for me to keep up in writing them down. I followed up my taste question by asking him about the smell and sound of poetry, and again he went into a deep concentration before the words flowed out in a torrent. Dr. London also shared with me how he feels people react to poetry.

This was on a Thursday. On Saturday, I got a call from Trudie telling me that her husband had died peacefully that morning. She wanted to know if I would send her the poem Dr. London and I had created. I typed up the poem from my notes to send to her.

I was honored to have spent time with Dr. London at the end of his life. His responses to my questions, which form the lines of the poem that follows, are in the order given, with light editing.

ON POETRY
DR. FRED LONDON

If I don't write it down, it's shhhhhhh.
Notice the color, this gray-brown
that eats up all the land.
When you reach out for it, it sneaks away.

Even though it sounds simple, it isn't simple—
It's like Frost, playing ball with a wasted arm.

A poem tastes sweet and orange flavored.
It grabs the poet by his trousers
and squeezes his crotch.
Stretching to gain more and he's lovable.

When you mention poetry to most people
they panic: smart people, dumb people.
I have no time for that.

Poetry smells like,
famine wolf-dog on a mountain,
running up the hill, biting the sun.

Once you read the poem,
you don't want to put it away.

Once the poem gets going—
you can actually miss tennis.

Poetry sounds like a howling wind,
pushing up the shore.

The Gathering Place

The Gathering Place is one of the best-organized adult day care centers I have worked with. They offer a range of art experiences, including working with concrete, which the men in the group really enjoy. Cindy Musial is the Executive Director. You can really see the spirit and sense of camaraderie she inspires in the participants. She is a true leader in the field. They have a one-to-one ratio of volunteers to people living with memory loss. It is to her credit that she inspires her community to such levels of support and involvement.

On a field trip to the John Michael Kohler Arts Center, I used the poem "Ocean" and the technique of asking open-ended questions to create a poem around the senses with the "poets" of The Gathering Place (see Ocean recipe that follows).

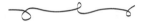

BON VOYAGE
JUDY PRESCOTT

Sometimes it's better to loosen
the spring line
and let her
float away.

If the storm is that great,
why keep her tethered,
battering herself to pieces
at the dock?

Let her go.
Watch her float peacefully away
under a grey and turbulent sky.

A last grand sail into
whatever lies beyond.

A graceful exit from all things
measured and charted.

Beautiful ketch,
I release you.

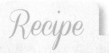 *Recipe*

DOCTOR LONDON'S LOVABLE LANGUAGE AU LAIT

INGREDIENTS:

1 bushel of poems (3 or more)
1 quiet room
1 comfortable place to sit
1 blank paper
1 writing utensil
2 people

INSTRUCTIONS:

Choose a bushel of poems with subject matter grouped around a theme. Perform the poems using call and response. You may gauge the participants' interest level. As they are still engaged in reciting the poems, gently shift from performing them to creating a poem together by asking opened-ended questions. Below is a typical progression of questions that you can use. Pick a theme and explore it through the participants' senses.

Would you like to create a poem together?

I am going to ask you questions about spring and write down your answers.

Your words will form the lines of the poem.

Shall we start?

continued

May I ask you a question, please?

We are going to create a poem about spring.

This is kind of a creative way to think.

What does spring taste like?

Imagine you are outside on a spring day.

What are the foods that make you think of spring?

What does spring smell like?

What does spring feel like?

What does spring sound like?

What does spring look like?

Continue to remind the participants that you are creating a poem to-gether based on spring, that you all are using your imagination and cre-ativity to talk about how spring tastes, looks, feels, sounds and smells. I recommend you emphasize to the group that their responses may be playful, silly, or even crazy!

After the poem has been created, you may perform it together to end the session. Thank everyone for their creativity.

OCEAN

INGREDIENTS:

1 life-size sculpture of a whale (or any artwork)
1 bucket of questions about oceans and whales
1 bushel of open minds and open ears
1 sack full of playful attitude with a pinch of sass
1 handful of being in the moment
1 gallon of open to where the poem takes you

INSTRUCTIONS:

I asked open-ended questions around the theme of whales and the ocean. As part of our field trip to the arts center, we were inspired by Tristin Lowe's sculpture *Mocha Dick*. The colossal sculpture is a 52-foot-long re-creation of the real-life albino sperm whale that terrorized early 19th-century whaling vessels near Mocha Island in the South Pacific. Mocha Dick, described in appearance as "white as wool," engaged in battle with numerous whaling expeditions and inspired Herman Melville's epic *Moby Dick*.

The open-ended questions I used included:

What do you think of when you hear the word *ocean*?

Does anyone like to go fishing?

What does the ocean sound like?

What does the ocean feel like?

What would you do if you saw a whale?

What would you say if you could speak to a whale?

continued

Here is a link to a performance of the poem we created: http://www. youtube.com/watch?v=Q4vFly6NuGQ

In the video of the performance you will see there was quite of bit of improvisation that influenced the structure and final text of the poem. When you are performing a poem with a group, be sure to also listen and allow space for spontaneous comments to become part of the poem. In the video, you will hear Nancy respond to the seagull sounds we are making with the lovely line, "And that's when the birds come." And at the end you will hear Olie finish the poem by playing off the rhyme "Pale whale ale" with the brilliant play on words "From a pail." Such moments are a large part of what makes the Alzheimer's Poetry Project thrive and garner robust responses.

Ocean Poem

The lake is fresh
The ocean is salt

It's so cold
When you're ice fishing
The fish don't smell
And that's why we ice fish

Ice fish
Ice fish
Nice fish

The ocean has quite a sound—
splashing, waves, and wind.

It can roar.

ROAR!

continued

Shhhhhhhhh . . . . .
Caw . . . caw . . . caw . . .

And that's when the birds come.

The ocean feels like foam—all the bubbles.

If a whale came along, I'd be scared.
If I could swim fast enough,
I'd get myself out of the water.

The whale is a something—BIG!

I wouldn't talk to a whale, unless I was formally introduced.

I would say to the whale, "Whale, do you have a problem?"

You know what I would say?
What would you say?

Shultz is my name!
What do you have to say to that, you big ole whale?
I'm not afraid of you.
With your blubber
And your tail
And your eating of . . . Kale.
And drinking of ale.
Whale ale!
Whale ale!
Pale whale ale!
From a pail!

On Chanting Poetry

Twenty thousand people are cheering, waves of shouts and applause are washing over us. The young poets are chanting:

Tyger, tyger burning bright!

The crowd is chanting along. This is the Precision Poetry Drill Team. The teenage poets are leaping up and down as if on pogo sticks. As their poetry coach, I spin and pump my fist, leaping about. For as far as we can see, the huge crowd of people, the length of three football fields, are cheering. This is a poetry dream come true. Performing at the Zozobra festival in Santa Fe, New Mexico, for this huge crowd of people has been one of the highlights of my life as a poet.

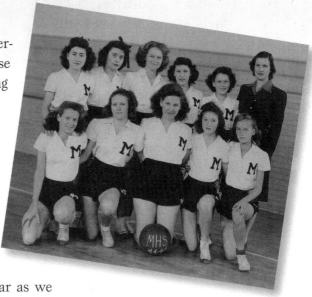

The concept of chanting a poem shifts the expectation of how poetry may be presented. It taps poetry at its roots as an oral art form. Chanting poetry opens up the performance of a poem to include cheerleading calls and military marching cadences.

I honed the technique of call and response during my work with the Precision Poetry Drill Team, working with middle and high school students as their poetry coach at Desert Academy in Santa Fe, New Mexico. We were featured on National Public Radio (http://www.npr.org/templates/story/story.php?storyId = 4615966).

Recipe

DELICIOUS TYGER PUNCH ·

INGREDIENTS:

1 poem (or select lines of poetry)
1 mouth (leader)
1 to 20,000 mouths (group)
1 smile

INSTRUCTIONS:

Below are the opening lines to William Blake's "The Tyger," which is quite fun to use. Shall we give it a go?

Tyger, tyger burning bright
In the forest of the night

say it softly.

Tyger, tyger burning bright
In the forest of the night

Say it loud.

Tyger, tyger burning bright
In the forest of the night

Say it in your natural speaking voice.

Tyger, tyger burning bright
In the forest of the night

Pep Talk
Repeat the opening lines with the group as necessary, to get the rhythm cooking: "Feel the sound shift in your head, throat, and body as you shift the volume. Now, try clapping along. If you are feeling playful, you can growl like a tiger at the end. Don't be afraid to be silly!"

continued

Below is the full poem for you to experiment with.

The Tyger
WILLIAM BLAKE

Tyger Tyger, burning bright,
In the forests of the night;
What immortal hand or eye,
Could frame thy fearful symmetry?

In what distant deeps or skies.
Burnt the fire of thine eyes?
On what wings dare he aspire?
What the hand, dare seize the fire?

And what shoulder, & what art,
Could twist the sinews of thy heart?
And when thy heart began to beat,
What dread hand? & what dread feet?

What the hammer? what the chain,
In what furnace was thy brain?
What the anvil? what dread grasp,
Dare its deadly terrors clasp!

When the stars threw down their spears
And water'd heaven with their tears:
Did he smile his work to see?
Did he who made the Lamb make thee?

Tyger Tyger burning bright,
In the forests of the night;
What immortal hand or eye,
Dare frame thy fearful symmetry?

Zozobra means *anxiety* in Spanish. As part of the festival, people are encouraged to write their "glooms" on a piece of paper that they then stuff into the 50-foot-tall effigy, so that their worries go up in smoke when the Old Man Gloom is burned.

The organizers had invited the Precision Poetry Drill Team to perform early in the event, and if they liked what we did they would invite us back to perform just before the burning of the effigy for the full audience.

The stage was on top of a hill at the end of a string of playing fields. We got to the concert early and performed for a few thousand people milling around and setting up blankets to settle in for the night. The organizers loved our performance and asked us to return at 9 p.m. to perform for the larger crowd.

My experience with the Precision Poetry Drill Team shows that using chanting when performing poetry has the potential to reach much larger audiences than a typical poetry reading.

Chanting Power

My first experience with the power of chanting was with junior high basketball and the cheerleaders calling out:

Gary, Gary, he's our man. If he can't do it, no one can. GO, GARY!

When I say those words using that school sports chant, the basketball court filled with fans shouting and pumping their fists in the air all comes back. The chant is powerful.

You can find inspiration for how to recite poetry from three very different groups—soldiers, cheerleaders, and monks.

Am I really suggesting you recite poetry while jumping around in a short skirt, waving pom-poms, and doing flips and cartwheels? Well, yes and no. I am really just encouraging you to think about the energy cheerleaders bring to leading the crowd. Is there anything there to inspire you in the way you say a poem? Consider military marching cadences. Not that you would recite a poem with such gusto, but the precision and power with which they chant the cadences might inspire you in how you say a poem. Regarding monks, I am thinking in particular of Gregorian chants. Many religions use chants in the pursuit of spiritual development, including Buddhism (chanting to prepare the mind for meditation), Judaism (cantillation), and Roman Catholicism (chanting of psalms).

This is a challenge to you, to expand the sound of the voice you think of when you think of a poem being recited.

SOME LIBRARIES
ZOË BIRD

I chose "The Library"
as theme for yesterday's poetry session
at the adult day center,
read Emily Dickinson, Charles Simic and Warren
leapt in immediately with a pun:
I guess,
if you have a doughnut,
you have a (w)hole
lot of flavor.

Shirl: I wish we could go back to Emily Dickinson's time
and sit with her, and watch her write poems.
And write poems the way she did.

Martha: No you don't! They had quill pens back then.
You had to dip and write, dip and write.
There were thousands of ink spills. Thousands! Poor lady.

Emily Dickinson's life was pretty sad in some ways, we agreed.
(Do they know she asked Sue to burn all the love letters?)

Robert: We went to a memorial for our friend yesterday.

Warren: It's like this sad story I read, Then Came Heaven.
The mother dies in an industrial accident,
the father blubbers into a towel at night

so the kids don't hear—
it was so sad
it made me want to play Hank Williams records for them.

The last song Hank Williams ever wrote
was "I'll Never Get Out of This World Alive."
It would be cool,
someone said,
if Emily Dickinson
could imagine an airplane.

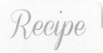

Recipe

FRESH HOT APPLE PIE, SMALL TOWN SCHOOL SPIRIT YELL

INGREDIENTS:

1 passel of cheerleaders
1 impressionable boy
1 sweaty school gym
35 years

INSTRUCTIONS:

This is your moment. You see the cheerleaders gathered by the bleachers. They are laughing and giggling. Their pom-poms are fluttering. They are chanting your name. Yes, here it comes: "Gary, Gary, he's our man. If he can't do it, no one can. Go, go, go, Gary!" You step to the free-throw line. You bounce the ball once. They chant your chant again. You steady the ball and keep your eyes on the rim of the basket. One more chant and you let fly the ball, your hand and arm following through with the arc of the ball, as if it were on a string and you could guide its flight. Then, swish. The ball goes perfectly through the hoop and net. The crowd explodes, and you hear them cheer.

Does the Monkey
Want a Peanut?

At one session in Georgia, I was reciting "The Tyger." I reached out my hand to a woman in the group to see if she would take it, and instead she looked at me and said, "Does the monkey want a peanut?" I'm reciting a 200-year-old poem—I do want a peanut! The woman spoke louder and louder, finally shouting, "Somebody get this MONKEY a peanut!" The nurses started laughing. I laughed as well and thought to myself that maybe the poetry program should be called the Alzheimer's Heckler Project.

Hammar, Götell, and Engström (2011) offer ways to handle situations such as the one during the session in Georgia. In their research paper "Singing While Caring for Persons with Dementia," they discuss how negatively expressed emotions and resistance may be decreased and positively expressed emotions increased when caregivers sing to a person with dementia. They describe in particular singing during morning care situations, such as dressing, brushing teeth or hair, and bathing or showering.

The caregivers were not trained singers. The idea in using singing is that anyone can try the technique. This was a single case study that included two women with severe dementia. Their resistance behavior during morning care situations included screaming or yelling and pulling away. When the caregivers engaged the women in singing, the negative behavior was reduced. This was a single case study with only a few people participating. With this in mind I want to expand our recipe repertoire.

One of the blessings in disguise in being a caregiver is you get to try new ideas. So pioneer, let's try this! I imagine you opening your mouth like an opera singer and belting out a resounding yeeeeessssss!

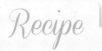

MONKEY WITH PEANUT SAUCE

INGREDIENTS:

1 poet dancing
1 woman yelling

INSTRUCTIONS:

Stir until thoroughly embarrassed

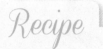

SPLISH, SPLASH

INGREDIENTS:

| 1 person | 1 caregiver |
| 1 song | 1 bath |

INSTRUCTIONS:

It is time for a bath or shower. You have the soap, towels, washcloth, and everything else you need ready. Pick one of the person's favorite songs. As you say to her gently, "Your bath is ready," begin to sing for her. See how she responds; does she sing along or just listen? Alternate singing with gentle instructions as you guide her to the bath or shower.

Is this approach working for you? For the person you are caring for? Is the morning ritual more joyful? This technique can be a way of reframing your attitude about a care task. It is common sense that if you are more relaxed, then the person you are caring for will be more relaxed. If you are smiling, it is more likely she or he also will be smiling.

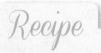
Recipe

BRUSH MY HAIR

INGREDIENTS:

2 people   1 brush

1 head of messy bed-head hair   1 rhythmic poem

INSTRUCTIONS:

It is time to wake up and smell the coffee, but first her hair could use a good brushing. Pick any poem, hopefully one with a strong rhythm. For this example, I suggest Robert Burns' "A Red, Red Rose."

As you say to her, "You have such lovely hair. May I please brush it for you?," begin to say the lines of the poem:

O my love is like a red, red rose
That's newly sprung in June:

Ask her if she would like to say the poem as well and, if so, have her repeat the words after you using the technique of call and response. Move the brush to the rhythm and speed you are using to brushing her hair. Say the next lines of the poem:

O my love is like a melody
That's sweetly played in tune!

You will need to practice saying the lines of the poem a few times until you can say them without looking at the written poem. You may, of course, have a copy of the poem with you. You do not want to be working without a net!

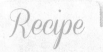

GIVE DANCE A CHANCE

INGREDIENTS:

2 people
2 shoes

INSTRUCTIONS:

The person you are caring for is bathed and her hair is brushed. She is ready to put her best foot forward and meet the day. In this exercise, you are going to make a game out of slipping the person's shoes on. I suggest you have her sit and then say, "Look, your shoes are dancing." You can playfully move the shoes in an imaginary dance. You can ask if she wants to see the shoes do a waltz or polka or for the shoes to do the twist.

Once you have set the tone that you are both having fun, sit across from or next to her so that she can see your feet and ask if she would also like to dance. Move your feet in a simple rhythm, perhaps just alternating left and right in a four-beat pattern, counting out, "One, two, three, four, one, two, three, four." Or perhaps you can hum a waltz and move your feet left and right, "One, two, three, one, two, three.

This exercise does not have to take much time, and shorter is probably better. Again, the goal is to reframe the care situation.

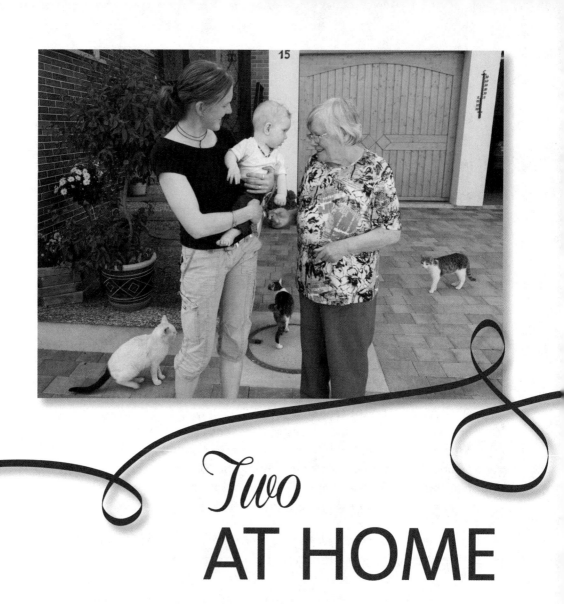

Two
AT HOME

Creating a Poem One-on-One and Using Large Type

We leaned in close to the tree and began to sniff. We inhaled the scent of the bark and looked at each other and laughed. It was silly and playful and a little bit weird, but also satisfying to get to know this tree through our senses. We felt the rough grain of the bark with our hands and the supple leaves as we rubbed them on our cheeks. We listened to the wind rush through the branches.

Working one-on-one with Karin Barreau in Madison, Wisconsin, has been one of my favorite experiences in creating poetry. Karin heard about the Alzheimer's Poetry Project through the Alzheimer's and Dementia Alliance of Wisconsin and arranged for me to visit her in her home to teach her some of our techniques. That was how I found myself with my nose pressed against her beloved tree.

We started the session by sitting together, talking, and sharing poems. I had brought a few poems with me that I printed with a large type size, so they might be easier to read. One of the poems was "Trees," by Joyce Kilmer, with its well-loved opening lines, "I think that I shall never see/a poem as lovely as a tree."

As we shared poems, I asked Karin if she wanted to try creating a poem together. I explained that I would ask her a series of questions and write down her answers and that they would become the lines of the poem. When I asked her what she wanted to write about, she said, "How about that tree in the front yard?"

We went outside and started by introducing ourselves to the tree! Karin and I created the poem that follows.

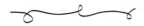

TREES

KARIN BARREAU

My favorite trees are many.
I love our tree out there.
I think it is a maple.
It smells soft
as washed clothes.
How high can you go up in a tree?
Feel the bark,
it has texture and feels heavy,
tastes icky,
looks beautiful.
The shape is beautiful,
a monument and a statue.
I can hear it talking.
I always hear trees talking.
Hello and welcome
and please do come sit
on me.

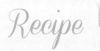

IF A TREE FALLS IN A FOREST . . .

INGREDIENTS:

Something to look at
2 curious minds
Something to write with
Something to write on
1 chunk of uninterrupted time (10 to 30 minutes)

INSTRUCTIONS:

With this recipe we look at creating a poem in a one-on-one setting. Choose something to look at and to write about. Some examples would be trees, flowers, animals, the sky, clouds, or children playing. Ask the person to describe what he or she is seeing. This works well if a room or location has a view. If it is nice weather, you might go outside for inspiration, as Karin and I did. Or you may try gathering a number of objects and having the person describe one.

TIPS ON CREATING A POEM TOGETHER:

Find a poem or a section of a poem that might be of interest to the person you are engaging with. Increase the font size of the text. Encourage the person to read the poem to you. Once you have had the person read the poem, you may try experimenting with having him or her lead you in call and response. Try this with a group of poems based on a theme.

Creating a Poem
Using Oral History

When Margaret and I sold the flower shop and traveled around the world for a year, one of the most interesting poets we met was Paul Polanski, who is best known for his work with the Roma, or Gypsy, people in Prague and the Czech Republic.

Polanski turns the oral history they share with him into poetry as a method of helping them share their story as a people, their experience during the Holocaust, and the discrimination they face today. Polanski has published 27 books, including 18 books of poetry and a number of nonfiction books. (You can read more about his work on his website [http://www.paul-polansky.nstemp.com].)

The following is the end of the poem "Grave Stones":

according to Romani tradition
the dead have no water in heaven
unless someone puts
two large river stones
on their grave

without stones
they have to beg for water
which is okay on earth

but not in heaven.

The Oral History Association website lists best practices and suggestions for what to do prior to taking an oral history, how to best conduct an oral history, and what to do after recording the oral history (http://www.oralhistory.org/about/principles-and-practices/). The association defines *oral history* as such:

a method of recording and preserving oral testimony and the product of that process. It begins with an audio or video recording of a first person account made by an interviewer with an interviewee (also referred to as *narrator*), both of whom have the conscious intention of creating a permanent record to contribute to an understanding of the past.

A verbal document, the oral history, results from this process and is preserved and made available in different forms to other users, researchers, and the public. A critical approach to the oral testimony and interpretations are necessary in the use of oral history.

In our work with people living with memory loss, I use the technique of recording an oral history and then turning it into a poem. I once recorded a conversation between Jose Mondragon, a resident of Sierra Vista Assisted Living Center, and me. During the interview, which happened spontaneously after a poetry session, I recorded Mr. Mondragon talking about an experience he had while working in a copper mine.

To create the poem, I transcribed Mr. Mondragon's interview. I then made some editing decisions about where to begin and end the poem. While I did not change any of the words, I did delete sections from the interview. This allowed for a process very similar to the creation of a poem through typical writing methods. I also made decisions about where to break the words into lines and how to shape the words on the page.

While we at the Alzheimer's Poetry Project are only beginning to use oral history tool to create poems, given the experience with Mr. Mondragon we are excited to explore this method, especially in the context of creating dementia-friendly communities and dementia-friendly businesses. Using oral history to create poems, stories, songs, and dances seems a natural extension of helping people become more aware of and engage with those living with memory loss.

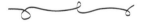

COPPER MINE
JOSE MONDRAGON

The rope was like a rope
you would tie a horse with,
about as thick as a quarter.
To pull you up or down
out of the mine.

The whole thing
came sliding down.
I put up my hands
against the board.

"Oh, God," that is all I say.

They tell me—
I don't see myself.

I was in a little hole
about as big as my body.

In the mine,
in the chute,
I held my breath.
I passed out.
They tell me—
I don't see myself.

A bunch of water,
blue, blue copper mining water,
it was running all around.
Dirt coming down the shaft.

That board came down.
I was standing to one side.
Looking up to the top.
Looking up to my partner.
I could see his light.

The dirt came down like snow.
I stuck my head underneath the board.

They put me on a stretcher
and brought me up the shaft.
They had one little cage.
It could hold only two men.
They put me in the cage,
standing straight up on the stretcher.

I passed out.
They took me to the hospital.

They put me in the hospital freezer—like I was dead.
I said, "God, help me."
They tell me—I never saw myself.

Everyday Speech as Poetry

When asked, people often say, "I don't know any poetry." Yet poetry is all around us, if you know where to look. For instance, have you ever felt "love at first sight"? That phrase comes from Christopher Marlow: "Love at first sight. Where both deliberate, the love is slight: Who ever loved, that loved not at first sight." How about the phrase "No man is an island"? That comes from a poem by John Donne. Below are both poems:

Who Ever Loved That Loved Not at First Sight?
CHRISTOPHER MARLOWE

It lies not in our power to love or hate,
For will in us is overruled by fate.
When two are stripped, long ere the course begin,
We wish that one should love, the other win;

And one especially do we affect
Of two gold ingots, like in each respect:
The reason no man knows; let it suffice
What we behold is censured by our eyes.
Where both deliberate, the love is slight:
Who ever loved, that loved not at first sight?

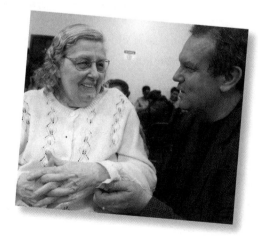

No Man Is An Island
JOHN DONNE

No man is an island,
Entire of itself,
Every man is a piece of the continent,
A part of the main.
If a clod be washed away by the sea,

Europe is the less.
As well as if a promontory were.
As well as if a manor of thy friend's
Or of thine own were:
Any man's death diminishes me,
Because I am involved in mankind,
And therefore never send to know for whom the bell tolls;
It tolls for thee.

Those phrases, which we have heard before and perhaps even used because we can relate to them, started as part of a poem. They have become so well known and used that they live in the rich world of our everyday language.

The website The Inky Fool ranks famous poetry lines by the number of times people search for them (http://blog.inkyfool.com/2012/01/fifty-most-quoted-lines-of-poetry.html). And, yes, Shakespeare by far has the most quotable lines, but surprisingly does not show up in the top ten.

Ranked number 27 is the quote that enticed thousands of women to join the Red Hat Society and to wear their striking purple outfits topped with jaunty red hats:

When I am an old woman I shall wear purple (Jenny Joseph)

At number 26 is the line of poetry I think is the most recognizable of any that I have used:

I think that I shall never see/A poem lovely as a tree (Joyce Kilmer)

Our dear Shakespeare's top entry is at number 13 with his parody of sonnets:

My mistress' eyes are nothing like the sun (Shakespeare)

Tennyson clocks in at number 10 with a line of poetry that has definitely crossed over into common usage:

Tis better to have loved and lost/Than never to have loved at all (Tennyson)

At number 3 is Wordsworth with:

The child is father of the man (Wordsworth)

Number two has the unfortunate and chilling distinction of having been chosen by Oklahoma City Bomber Timothy McVeigh as part of his last words upon his execution:

I am the master of my fate (William Ernest Henley)

Like with David Letterman reading his top ten list, you can almost feel the drum roll as we announce the number 1 most quoted line of poetry. In fact, why not say it to someone today:

To err is human; to forgive, divine (Alexander Pope)

Outside of poetry we have wonderful phrases such as "Forget about it!" and "How sweet it is!" There is the famous Yogi Berra quote, "It ain't over till it's over." The job of the adman is to create phrases that will stick in our heads, such as "It takes a licking and keeps on ticking" and "A little dab'll do ya." And then there are proverbs and sayings such as: "A stitch in time saves nine," "An ounce of prevention is worth a pound of cure," "A rolling stone gathers no moss," or Abraham Lincoln's pithy "In the end, it's not the years in your life that count. It's the life in your years."

These chunks of language can be fun to talk about and share. They can lead us to other memorable quotes, much like eating potato chips ("Bet you can't eat just one").

It is interesting to note that often when we remember a phrase we tend to know the whole phrase. If you start to say a phrase and a person has heard it before and knows it, he or she is able to finish the phrase. This can be a pleasurable activity that you can turn into a game.

Recipe

FANNIE FARMER'S FESTIVAL OF WORDS

INGREDIENTS:

1 level head
2 pecks of listening ears
10 famous quotes

INSTRUCTIONS:

Write down about 10 quotes. Share these examples with the group and ask the participants what other quotes come to mind. Ask the group to think of famous lines from movies. Are there phrases that the participants always say, or that people in their lives say? Perhaps something a parent or teacher always said?

Talk about the phrases: What do they convey? What emotions or thoughts do they elicit? Is there a power in such phrases? Are they funny? What makes them memorable? How do clichés become clichés?

Does the group know these phrases? Are there famous lines from poems that come to mind for the group? How do lines from poems become well-known phrases?

Use the poem "I'm Nobody!" by Emily Dickinson, with its delightful line, "I'm nobody, who are you?" Talk about the contrast between being nobody and being famous. What benefits are there to being unknown? To being known? What are the qualities that make a phrase famous? A person?

Write down the responses, which will become the lines of the poem. End the session with a call-and-response performance of the new poem.

Alternatively, a "found" poem can be created by writing the responses down in the order they are given, and then this list of sentences becomes the poem. The workshop can end with a group reading of the poem or poems created.

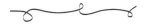

FOREVER INTO CONSTELLATIONS
JOANNE DWYER

We were handed sunlight and the smooth landing of leviathan
white-winged birds on our tongues and on our back porches.

We were given a sky that would shelter us from falling debris
and eyes that could see forever into constellations.

We never imagined a day we would not know the names of the
babies we birthed and the husbands and wives with whom we

shot arrows, danced, skinned fish and bought patio furniture.
We were of the belief that our bones would never be as brittle

as moth wings; our lungs as narrow a passage as plastic straws.
We were gifted tower-tall verdant and sinuous stalks of corn

on which to climb as sure-footed as fur-matted mountain goats
from which to gaze the far world and foresee any fires or

thunderous herds of caribou—and call out a credible warning.
We were given hands that could forever knit caps in the colors

of incarnadine and copper; mouths that could forever name
the fruits falling from our trees and berries landed in our laps.

We never imagined a day we would not know the meaning of
such words as *venison* or *duck; marble cake* or *mudpie.*

We could never have been prepared for the receding waters
vacating us and the power lines never being repaired.

At first, the tunnels seemed like paper; later they became brick.
And our practiced tongues became artifacts under sand.

Obscured night arrives like a hood thrown over our heads. And
we walk uneasily into it, with hands outstretched like the blind.

And learn to lean into the dark, as if into the wind, as if leaning
on the arm of a massive and constant god in a long wool coat.

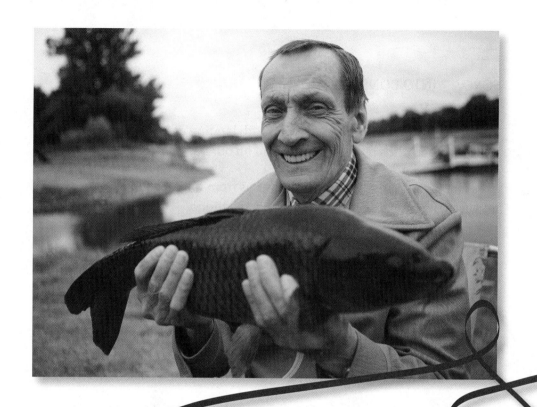

Three
CAREGIVER WRITING PROMPTS

The Ballad of
the Happy Guitar
How to Write a Letter Poem

After giving a poetry reading in Appleton, Wisconsin, and speaking about the Alzheimer's Poetry Project, the writer Abby Frucht came up and spoke to me about her mother who had Alzheimer's disease and how hard it was that her mother was living in an assisted living center. I asked if her mother was near Appleton, thinking perhaps I could go and work with her. She said no, that her mother was living in Santa Fe at Sierra Vista. I then shared with her that I had started the Alzheimer's Poetry Project in Santa Fe, and that Sierra Vista was the first place where I had worked. Abby described her mother, and I realized that I knew her, that she was in a recent group I had worked with. I offered to share with Abby the poem her mother's group had created. I sent her the poem and both she and her sister guessed correctly that the line their mother contributed was, "I'd find that very hard."

That day when I had worked with the group at Sierra Vista, Joan Logghe, the Santa Fe poet laureate, joined in with her class from the Santa Fe Girls School. Our model poem was "A Red, Red Rose," by Robert Burns. The group asked a series of questions around the theme of love. The participants' responses form the lines of the poem on the page that follows.

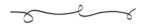

LOVE POEM

How do I express my love?
With feeling

Love is one of the most
tender things we have.
Love is a strong scent.

I'd find that very hard.

It can be as simple as—I love you.
That's it.

I love you very, very much.
I love you, too, my husband.

I love you like a red, red, rose.

I think it is nice to be with this group here.

Does love have deep issues?
I'm scared. I'm tired.

When I was in nurses training I had a maid; she called me.
She said, "Your boyfriend Robbie Burns is here!"

I love you.

I always say, if the coat is on sale, get it!
I got the green one, but I really liked the blue one.

I am very honored with many friends and family,
who are kind and loving to me.

I love you-u-u-u-u.

Abby called me not long after sharing the poem with her to say that Sierra Vista had asked her if she would stop calling her mother, that her mother no longer recognized who was calling and that the calls were causing her to feel disoriented and upset. That, of course, is one of the worst things that family members have to deal with; that is, the point in the disease process where their loved one no longer remembers who they are. I cannot imagine a more painful experience. Abby asked if I had any suggestions. I encouraged her to write something for her mother and that I would share it with her mother the next time I worked at Sierra Vista. Abby composed a poem in the form of a letter, recalling a much happier time:

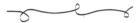

DEAR MOM,

I remember a song called
"The Sad Guitar."
You sang it
to Sylvia and Liz and Me
when we were little girls.
We loved it.
You strummed it for us
on an air guitar
whenever we wanted
to hear it.
The guitar was sad
but you make us happy.

Love,
Abby

Our model poem for the next workshop at Sierra Vista was "The Owl and the Pussy Cat," with its wonderful line "the owl looked up to the stars above and sang to a small guitar." We took our cue from Abby's poem, and while performing the poem we all strummed imaginary "air guitars." I kneeled by her mother and chanted the end of the poem:

. . . hand in hand on the edge of the sand
we danced by the light of the moon . . .

. . . the moon, the moon, the moon
we danced by the light of the moon.

I took her hands and moved them to the rhythm of the poem, creating a sort of dance between us. I moved around the room and asked each person if they also wanted to feel the rhythm of the poem. It was joyful and felt like we were having a party. People were laughing and chanting along with the poem. At moments like that, with the room full of people smiling and laughing, it feels like there is no dementia in the room.

We created the following poem by asking the participants what makes them happy. Abby's mother's line in this poem is, "When I am feeling well and I have good people with me, that makes me happy."

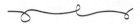

THE BALLAD OF THE HAPPY GUITAR

A happy guitar,
with my husband.
Everything makes me happy.
Anyone makes me happy.
To dance makes me happy.
The Owl and the Pussy Cat!
Having you here.
It's nothing immediate.
The sound of a mandolin
makes me happy.
My father played
the mandolin.
I want to dance some more!
When I am feeling well
and I have good people with me,
that makes me happy.

MS. ABBY FRUCHT'S HEIRLOOM LETTER POEM

INGREDIENTS:

2 hearts
1 pure, white blank page (or more)
1 heaping helping of desire to communicate
1 ink bottle (midnight black)
1 quill pen (or ball-point pen, if quill is unavailable)
1 writing desk (cherry and black walnut roll-top, if possible)
1 oil lamp (or well-stoked brick fireplace)
1 hand-sewn quilt to place on lap (optional)
1 parlor

INSTRUCTIONS:

Now that you have re-created a nineteenth-century writing room, you are ready to write. Or, more likely, if you are like me, you have pushed back clutter from the kitchen table and cleared an open space for your note-book. This writing prompt is simple. Think of someone you love and write a letter to that person. Or take a page from the great American songbook and do as Joe Young describes in his famous lyrics: "I'm gonna sit right down and write myself a letter and make believe it came from you."

Either way you are connecting with your loved one and using the form of a letter to write to him or her and to imagine he or she is writing to you. Imagine the person's face as you write. Imagine you are speaking directly to your loved one and how he or she would respond. This could be a real letter you put a stamp on to mail to your loved one or an imaginary letter you mail from your heart.

Lucile

On Creating a Poem Using a Timed Writing Exercise

One person I really enjoyed working with was Lucile Adler. Lucile was a poet, who had been published by *The New Yorker* and *Poetry* magazines. She also published an anthology titled *Amulet Songs: Poems Selected and New*. She had a great knowledge of poetry and loved Yeats. She organized poetry readings and published local poets in poetry magazines. In essence, Lucile was a poetry mover and shaker.

Her family had learned of the APP and asked if I could work with her. She was living at Aspen Ridge Lodge in Los Alamos, New Mexico. I arranged to visit her with her daughter.

As everyone gathered for the poetry session in the common area, I held up Lucile's book and said, "I want to share poetry with you today." Lucile said, "I have a book just like that in my room." "This is your book, Lucile, and these are your poems. Today we are going to hear work from William Shakespeare, William Blake, Edgar Allen Poe, and Lucile Adler." The group was fascinated that they had a published poet living with them.

As I was reciting the opening couplet from Blake's "The Tyger," she said, "You know that poem has more than two lines." She challenged me to see if I could recite the whole poem, and when I finished she said, "Oh, so you do know it."

After the session, Lucile, her daughter, and I went to Lucile's room. We read poems by Yeats and I pointed out places in her poems where I thought Yeats might have influenced her poetry. It was a delightful afternoon.

Sometime later I learned that the week before Lucile passed away she kept telling everyone she was going on a trip. The morning she passed away, Lucile took her purse and gathered up items you might take on a trip. She then sat on the couch in the common area, flipped her scarf over her neck, and died. Here is a section from Lucile's poem, "Red Shoes Dancing":

To be old and to have joined others who are old
In an Old People's home
Is perhaps the least distinguished stay
Of a lifetime—certainly the loneliest

At the time of writing the poem, Lucile was living in an assisted living center. She perfectly captures that emotional experience. She also turns the lonely, "least distinguished stay" on its head and finds a way to triumph:

God, forgive those of us who rebel
And resist in red shoes
By dancing wildly below a cold sky

In the last lines of the poem she combines the loneliness with her rebellion in this beautiful stark image:

Dancing alone
From now on . . .

It was such a pleasure to get to know and work with Lucile. Consider her idea of rebellion as a theme for writing a poem. How would you, as a caregiver, rebel? As a healthcare professional, how would you rebel?

The writing prompt recipe featured in this chapter is based on the concept of continuous writing. I was introduced to this technique in 7th grade. Each afternoon the teacher would have us write on any topic. The only rule was not to stop writing. I think she did this because we were a noisy, unruly class and this was a way to maintain control of us and make us work.

One benefit of writing nonstop for a period time is that it turns off your inner editor, the little voice that tells you as you are writing "this is no good," that thinks of spelling and grammar, that worries about what people will think when they read what you have written. As a poet, you, of course, may always choose to write about any subject; the writing idea with this exercise, however, is to be inspired by Lucile. She rebelled against the "Old People's home" by dancing.

The following recipe encourages the participants to consider what they would rebel against. Ask the group "What form will your rebellion take?" Tell them that this is their chance to express their frustrations, to list their complaints, to, yes, bitch and moan. Lucile did not just dance; she danced in "red shoes." Ask the participants to think about what object(s) would assist them in their rebellion.

Recipe

LUCILE'S FRESH BLANK PAPER
WITH VERY HOT INSPIRATION

INGREDIENTS:

1 writing *utensil*
1 blank page
2 dollops of imagination
10 minutes (or more)
1 comfortable place to sit
1 quiet room or, alternatively, 1 noisy coffee house

INSTRUCTIONS:

This is will be a performance served up in a loose sense of the word. You will write for 10 minutes without stopping. Your performance will be keeping your pen moving, no matter what.

RECOMMENDATIONS:

The most famous proponent of timed writing exercises is Natalie Goldberg, author of the hugely popular book *Writing Down the Bones: Freeing the Writing Within*, which offers many detailed writing prompts and exercises.

Listening as Poetry
How to Write an "I Hear" Poem

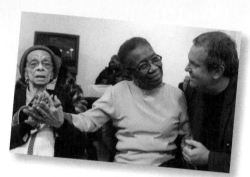

In a very real sense, the job of being a poet is to write down what you hear around you and sometimes what you hear in your head. As a prompt to help get you started on writing for this exercise, begin by taking a walk. Listen and write down what you hear.

You will write a poem for this exercise, but you will not worry about rhyme or rhythm; you will just write down what you hear and use what you have written down to create an "I hear" poem.

Time to get out your caregiver notebook and a pen. You do have a caregiver notebook, don't you? You should have a little blank book to write down your thoughts and questions. Things you want to remember while caregiving and having a little book allows you to keep them in one place and to be able to find them easily.

Take a walk, notice the sounds you hear, and write them down. That will be your poem for today.

Here is an "I hear" poem I wrote for you:

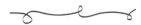

I HEAR POEM
GARY GLAZNER

I hear the rain, wet and slapping on the sidewalk.
The sound is running down from the roof,
into the gutter, wet and happy.
It sounds like laughter
I hear the sound of my umbrella opening.
The sound is how I imagine a parachute sounds,
when opening, all at once,

and it makes me feel safe.
I hear the raindrops falling on my umbrella.
Gene Kelly, anyone?
I hear far in the distance, the hum of car wheels on the road.
I hear my shoes, on the pavement.
I hear a bird, chirping.
I stop and hear that everything is quiet,
except for the rain.
I hear a building humming, a generator song.
I hear more birds join in
to form a bird chorus.

As I listen, I feel myself being fully in the moment or simply paying attention. My mind feels refreshed by my walk. As I listen to the sounds around me and I write them down, I might find my thoughts drifting to my loved one and write those down as well. For me, and I hope for you, I find what a pleasure it is to be a caregiver, and even though it is the hardest thing I have ever done in my life, it is such an honor.

A Word on Silence and John Cage

The composer John Cage was famous for his 1952 composition 4'33", which is remarkable in that the musicians who present the work play no music, but only sit silently for the length of time specified by the title.

Often they come out into the concert hall, flip up the tails of their tuxedos, sit down at or with their instrument, and then remain motionless for exactly 4 minutes and 33 seconds. They they rise, bow, and walk off the stage, with another grueling performance behind them.

As they sit there, you as the audience start to become aware of the sounds in the concert hall—shuffling feet, coughing, traffic seeping in from outside, your breathing. It is unsettling and makes you think about silence and what sounds we are always awash in as we go about our day.

Cage once said, "The sound experience which I prefer to all others, is the experience of silence. And this silence, almost anywhere in the world today, is traffic. If you listen to Beethoven, it's always the same, but if you listen to traffic, it's always different."

Cage had a favorite habit of wishing people, "Happy New Ears."

So, here's to you! Cheers! Wishing you Happy New Ears!

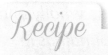

JOHN CAGE'S HAPPY NEW EAR STEW WITH PAY ATTENTION GRAVY

INGREDIENTS:

1 caregiver notebook
1 writing utensil
1 chunk of time (10 minutes? 15 minutes? Half an hour? A whole hour!)
A pair of comfortable shoes
A place to walk

INSTRUCTIONS:

Put on your shoes, get your notebook and pen, set aside a little time for yourself, and take a walk. As you walk, pay attention to the sounds around you and write them down. Have fun! Think of yourself as a poetry reporter and the sounds are the story you are reporting on. Slow down and listen to all of the sounds around you.

That absorption in the moment—that being so wholly and utterly carried away and inspired by the surroundings in which one happens to be—what can one do about it? And even if one could resist it if one wanted to, what would be the point, why shouldn't one give oneself over to that which is in front of one, as this, after all, is the surest way to create something?

—VINCENT VAN GOGH, IN A LETTER TO THEO VAN GOGH (1888)

Main Street as Poetry
How to Write an "I See" Poem

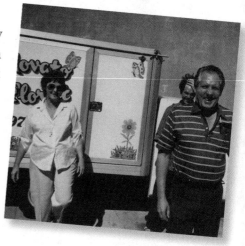

During all of the years I worked as a florist, my favorite job was sweeping the sidewalk out in front of the store. The street was called Grant Avenue and it was a classic small town main street. When I would arrive to the store early in the morning before the rest of the staff, it was quiet. I would start my day by sweeping off the sidewalk. I felt like the sheriff of Main Street—protective, in charge, and in control. Whatever the rest of the day would bring, that was a moment of peace.

For this exercise, I hope you will feel a moment of peace and control. This is a simple activity built on taking a walk. Depending on where you live, you might start by taking a walk around your neighborhood.

Bring your caregiver notebook and pen with you. Open up the door and off you go! As you walk along, slow down and look around you. Maybe even before you step out, take a deep breath and center yourself.

Stop along the way and write down what you notice. It does not have to be elaborate or fancy. Jot down a simple description of something that catches your eye. Do not worry about rhyming or rhythm. Describe things you see that are interesting to you. This type of poem is called a "list" poem, or an "I see" poem.

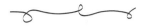

NOVATO
GARY GLAZNER

I see the sidewalk is covered with seedpods
dropped from the Liquid Amber trees.
They are spiny little balls

as if a golf ball had mated with a porcupine.
I see the flower shop window has a back-to-school display
with giant crayon and a blackboard
that says welcome back.
I see the jewelry store display is full of diamond rings
and photographs of happy just married couples.
I see the shoe repair store and hear its machines whirring.
I see the candy store; it is pulling at me like a magnet
to go in and let my sweet tooth have its way.
I see the bookstore with a cat in the window guarding
all that knowledge.
I see the sporting goods store
Its window full of balls, bats, gloves, and childhood dreams.

You can see in my poem that I use the phrase "I see" to give a little shape
to the poem and as a launching pad for my observations. After each "I see"
line, I give a brief description of and context to what I was seeing. You may
try that as well or just stick with describing what you saw. Alternatively,
you could use your imagination to visit a street from your childhood or from
some other time in your life. Or even expand on the idea and take an imaginary visit to a street from the old west or the Middle Ages, or even write a
description of a street on a far away distant planet. It is your choice; after all,
you are the poet!

Bonus: Poet as Reporter

Along your walk you may encounter people and stop to speak with them.
Consider including them in the poem. For fun, if you feel comfortable, you
may even say, "Hey, I'm writing a poem. Do you want to be in it?" You could
ask the person to tell you something he or she finds interesting along the
street, or something funny that happened on the street. Now you are poet
and reporter! Use the person's responses to create the poem.

Recipe

THE BOY FLORIST'S STATE FAIR, BLUE RIBBON, MAIN STREET, MAIN DISH

INGREDIENTS:

1 caregiver notebook
1 writing utensil
1 chunk of time (10 minutes? 15 minutes? Half an hour? A whole hour!)
A pair of comfortable shoes
A place to walk

INSTRUCTIONS:

Put on your shoes, get your notebook and pen, set aside a little time for yourself to take a walk. As you are walking, pay attention to the sights around you and write them down. Have fun! Think of yourself as a poetry reporter and the sights are the story you are reporting on. Slow down and open your eyes to all of the colors, images, and people around you.

You will notice this is the same recipe as "Listening as Poetry," with looking replacing *listening* as the main activity. Hopefully both recipes will inspire you to be more aware. In paying attention to the details of life, we want to replenish ourselves and bring that renewal to our tasks as caregivers as well as to taking care of ourselves.

Work as Poetry

For this activity, the idea is to create a poem using the theme of work. Working with Dr. Peter Reimann and his daughter, Hannah, in Springfield, New Jersey, we created a poem based on his responses to the question "What does it mean to be a doctor?"

Dr. Reimann is very playful and freely makes up rhymes. He jokes that his name means "rhyming man." He knows many German poems by heart and recited and translated a few for us on the spot. Hannah wrote down his responses to create the lines of the poem and translated the German lines.

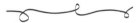

WHAT DOES IT MEAN TO BE A DOCTOR?
DR. PETER REIMANN

What it means to be a doctor
is a number of things.
People come to you
and want advice about their health
and they complain about what they consider
is missing from their health
Or they don't.
They say, "What the hell do you think is wrong with me?
Lass mich allein, I'm fine
und du bist für mich ein Borstenschwein!"*

What advice would I give a young doctor?
First, I'd ask, "Why do you want to be a doctor?
Is it that you want to make money?
What for?
Or is it that you want to help other people?
What fur?"

You ask me what was my reason to be a doctor.
I think my question was something of natural history.
Why are there people who need help?
Very complex, of course.
Do they need help because
of the hostile environment
or their internal hostility
or blah, blah, blah

What was the best thing about being a doctor?
. . . okay, one more question: $10—
Another complex question.
It's a job in which you keep your hands clean
You don't get literally dirty
or it's a job in which you make people feel a little better
or you make them feel really bad
Is that good?
Could be good—
Could be really bad . . .
and so on
and so on

*Translation: "Leave me alone, I'm fine.
and you are for me a pig with many stiff hairs in his snout!"*

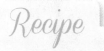
Recipe

WORKING WOMAN STEW WITH A SIDE OF CRUSTY WORKING MAN BREAD

INGREDIENTS:

1 lifetime of work
1 comfortable place to sit
1 curious person
1 worker

INSTRUCTIONS:

Start by asking the group what they did for work or still do for work. Did they enjoy their work? Do they still enjoy working? Once the conversation starts to progress, the participants may talk freely about where they used to work or the different jobs they had. They may even talk about work they still do. Working in the garden. Making meals for family and friends. Explore with the group what it means to work. Write down their responses. Perform the poem with the group using call and response, or perhaps have them read you the finished poem.

Bonus

You may want to share your work experiences as well.

Creating with a Family Member

If your are engaging a family member in this activity, you might start by talking about how much you appreciate the work he or she did and explore with the person what he or she enjoyed about working. That can then lead into creating the poem about their work.

Esther's Caregiver Writing Workshop

Poet Esther Altshul Helfgott is the author of *Dear Alzheimer's: A Caregiver's Diary & Poems*, which chronicles her experience caring for her husband, Abe Schweid. She also writes the blog, "Witnessing Alzheimer's: A Caregiver's View," for the SeattlePI.com reader (http://blog.seattlepi.com/witnessingalzheimers/). Esther has also taught writing workshops for caregivers as a way for participants to share their unique stories and to help them understand and cope with the many thoughts and feelings that come into play in caring for someone with Alzheimer's or related dementias.

An Interview Esther Altshul Helfgott

(Gary) What is the inspiration behind teaching a class for caregivers?

(Esther) I've been teaching people who care for others for many years, either in senior adult education programs, where the participants were mostly women who had spent a lifetime taking care of their families, or at Cancer Lifeline, where participants were caring for themselves, parents, siblings, or partners. So it's been a natural progression for me to want to put skills I've already developed to work in the field of Alzheimer's caregiving, although some in my current class are caring for people who have Parkinson's or another form of debilitating disease. Caregiving is caregiving, so I open the class to everyone, although, to be sure, Alzheimer's has its own specificities. Still it's good, I think, for caregivers of "different persuasions" to hear each other's stories. It puts us on the same platform, says we all have hardships to deal with in our daily lives or, in some cases, years.

(Gary) What do you hope to achieve with the class?

(Esther) I hope to create a circle of caregivers who meet in community to discuss the ups and downs of the caregiving experience. To help people not

feel so alone in the isolation that caregiving often brings about. To use writing as a tool to help caregivers understand their thoughts and feelings about the roles they are in. To use writing as a way to make it through the day. Everyone can write, and everyone's story is important to record, so we as a civilization understand the throes and nuances of the human condition. Writing brings one closer to the self and the self's experience with the other, so it is most important to develop as a personal learning tool. I hope to help people learn to use writing to understand the dynamics they are experiencing when interacting with others, whether within the caregiving community or beyond. That said, my focus is on developing class participants as writers. While they write about personal problems, I always suggest seeking out a social worker or therapist to resolve them.

(Gary) How do you structure the workshop?

(Esther) My workshops are structured organically. My first job is to get everyone to begin to know each other. On the first day, we go around the room and tell our stories. If the class is too big for a 2-hour session, I break up into twos and have participants interview each other. Then they come back to the group and introduce their partner to the whole group. I may have them write about the experience afterwards or take an idea or sentence or word that they've heard in the go-around, something that especially touched them, and write about it on the page (we don't use computers; I find them very distracting). I ask them to free associate, write whatever comes to mind, without editing yourself or worrying about spelling or grammar.

For years, I taught a class called "Poeming the Silence," in which I used poems as triggers for writing exercises, but even in those classes and workshops I don't ask people to write in poem or any specific form. I ask participants to write in whatever way the words fall out of their pens: lists, circles, names of people/places, fantasies, life story, current story. Whatever comes to mind.

In my current caregiving class, for one exercise I hid a little poetry in my instructions. For instance, write four paragraphs/stanzas with only four lines each. Then find a title to what you've written. They had no idea they were writing poems!

(Gary) Please share a sample lesson or writing prompt you have used.

(Esther) One writing prompt uses collage. I like to combine writing with art, so at the end of a session I gave the following homework assignment: (1) photocopy a piece of the writing you did in class today. (2) Cut out words, sentences, or ideas that have special meaning for you. Lay them aside. (3) Cut out pictures from magazines or photos you especially like from your photo

albums—but scan them into your computer first! Paste them onto a canvas (cardboard, political sign you still have lying around from the last election, scrap of wood, cereal box, etc.), and make a design for yourself. Intersperse words and pictures to make a new story and more stories, if you like.

Everyone brought in a collage. I was especially impressed with one woman who used fabric to display her pictures. Sewing, knitting, and such are fields we can draw on to integrate with our writing lives. Who doesn't have scraps of material around, hooks and eyes, needles, pins. I still have my mother's dressmaking scraps.

Another prompt involves bringing in a photo of when you were a small child. Bring one in which you are smiling. Now that you are in the caregiving role, can you remember yourself at that time? Please write what comes to mind. This is an amazing exercise. You would be surprised at what comes out, tears but also laughter, with others in the group, everyone laughing together. People come in sad and go home with a little bit of smile in their faces.

(Gary) Any tips you would give someone who wants to teach a writing workshop for caregivers?

(Esther) I've often thought I need to keep my writing self outside of the workshop, that reading my own work takes students' time away; but in a class for caregivers of people with Alzheimer's, it seems especially important for me to share my writing experiences with the group. "We want to know you," a participant once said to me. She had been to one of my *Dear Alzheimer's* readings and was so pleased to know my story. In class that week she said: "Will you read what you've written today?" And, of course, I did and continue to do so in this particular class.

Don't be afraid to show your vulnerability. Listen carefully to what participants are saying. Be in their moment, not yours (as you would for an Alzheimer's patient), all the while keeping order and structure so the class can proceed on schedule.

(Gary) Anything else you care to add?

(Esther) A newspaper editor asked me what writing my book has meant to me. This is what I told her. It may be helpful for your book as well.

Writing *Dear Alzheimer's: A Caregiver's Diary & Poems* has given me the opportunity to reach a broad spectrum of people who are touched by Alzheimer's disease and other dementias. It has helped me understand the complexities involved in caregiving and the complications that caregiving brings to relationships, not just to the immediate and extended family, but to relationships in general. While writing the book has brought me closer to the caregiving experience, it has also separated me from it, since the book now feels as if it has a life of its own, has its own personhood and that it lives apart from me and Abe. Most of all, writing the book has meant a broadening of my community; it has allowed me to open a window to a world of differences.

I was in a poetry therapy workshop some years ago. We were asked to interview the person sitting next to us. Here's the poem I came up with, practically already finished inside my pen:

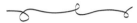

SERENDIPITY AT A POETRY THERAPY WORKSHOP:
WE'RE INSTRUCTED TO INTERVIEW THE PERSON SITTING NEXT TO US
(for Norma Leedy, and in memory of Jack Leedy,
founder of the National Association of Poetry Therapy)

There must have been
an angel
sitting here
between us
waiting for our pens
to meet
over husbands'
slipping minds.

Jack's
forty-five years
of patients
and poetry.

Abe's
forty-five years
of oncology and
microscopes
cell after cell
of stunning
destruction

Two doctors' wives
reeling.

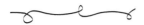

DEAR ALZHEIMER'S:

Why
did you pick our
sheltered
lives
to
visit?

An excerpt from *Dear Alzheimer's:*

April 6, 2007

Can we meet for dinner, he asks when I call at 4:50, right before his sup-per hour. It doesn't matter that I was there yesterday and we loved as we could love.

I know I shouldn't ask him, "Do you remember I was there yesterday? but I forgot and ask him anyway and thus I speak more of me than of him.

My words roll right by us as he asks again, Can we meet for dinner?

I am shamed back into his reality and say to him, "Tomorrow, tomorrow for lunch, we'll meet tomorrow for lunch." He is more than satisfied, says, "That will be just fine. What time should we get together?" as if he's ask-ing for a date. I say, "I'll pick you up at noon" and he says "I'll try to make it." Is he playing hard to get? Is he? How can the heart not break?

There are those who say: "You're not getting anything back. You need to move on and find a new life for yourself." And I wonder why they think I don't get anything back when learning Alzheimer Speak is as good as going for another Ph.D. Or looking in the mirror. To find myself inside the other.

April 9, 2007

I miss me,
    he said.
I miss you too

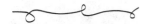

THREE CHILDHOOD POEMS IN WINTER
For Wilder's Great Room

RACHEL MORITZ

I.

The curved fenders of Model T's
are not the image your words give
but the shape drifting around them:

"I was born in Chicago in 1924."

Lake gusts, cranking radiators,
oilcloth table by kerosene light.
The doctor leaves your mother's bedroom
and behind his back, as the door clicks shut,
she gives you a different name.

II.

The light in winter is dull and sometimes sad.
There are paper birds tethered to strings above our heads.
Our nametags clip smartly to wool collars and fleece.
We are finding words like dipping our hands in a pail of water.

III.

What country am I living in:
"Middle age"

What country am I living toward:
"Old age"

What country is the bright realm of childhood
tethered already in time's holding net:

"We pulled the figs off trees in our front yard"
"when I was five, in Mississippi"

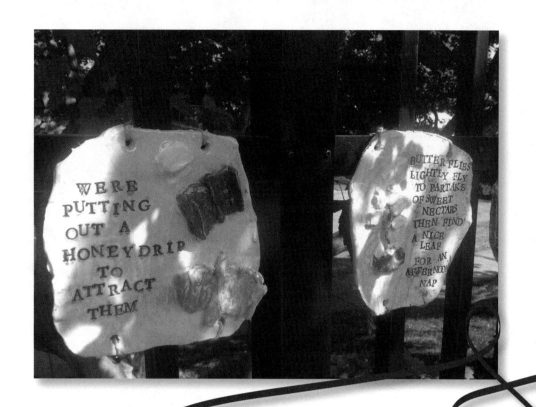

Four
ART

Art Inspiring the Performance and Creation of Poetry

A step away from the Vincent van Gogh painting *The Starry Night,* gesticulating wildly, I led twenty people living with dementia and their care partners in a group performance of our newly created poem inspired by this masterpiece.

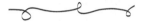

STARRY NIGHTS

Appreciative.
Very calm—and yet there's turmoil.
A little suspect, a little sinister,
something evil about it, that plant.
Confusing.

A star tastes delicious.
A star tastes like a milky way.

If I had a thought, I would but you're okay
so you can get away.

A star smells like peanut butter.
You've got to do it!

The stars sound like full heritage.
Everyone looks at a star and dreams.

A star sounds like a symphony.

The painting is soothing, you could sleep happily.
I see bipolar, I feel pity for the person
describing his feelings in the painting.

You can read a lot into Van Gogh's painting.

I like the sun, the way it moves.
Oh, my goodness!
Let me think about that now.

Not to count everything that you can use.

It looks like a storm.
Blue is his favorite color—as we can see.

Francesca Rosenberg, Director of Community, Access, and School Programs in the Department of Education at MoMA, knew of my work with the Alzheimer's Poetry Project and had invited me to co-lead a session of "Meet Me at MoMA." This innovative arts program is open to people living with Alzheimer's disease and their families once a month. The idea for our session using *The Starry Night* was to blend the techniques Rosenberg and MoMA's staff have developed in providing intimate gallery tours for people navigating Alzheimer's and their families with the APP method of performing and creating poetry—using the art as inspiration.

We began the MoMA session with Alberto Rios's "Museum Heart," a poem that celebrates museums. Using the technique of call and response, we performed the opening lines:

We, each of us, keep what we remember in our hearts.
We, all of us, keep what we remember in museums.
In this way, museums beat inside us.

Francesca and I led the group in perhaps MoMA's first art cheer, a rousing chant of: Picasso! Rousseau! Go van Gogh!

I chose Picasso's *Les Demoiselles d'Avignon* (*The Young Ladies of Avignon*) to begin the tour. One way to pair poetry and art is to use poetry created by the artist. In researching the curriculum, I had learned that from 1935, when Picasso was 54, until 1959 he wrote poetry on a regular, often daily, basis.

It is now part of the Picasso myth that in 1935, for the first time in his life, he stopped making art for a year and began writing poetry because he was going through a divorce. The theory is Picasso did not want any newly created art to become part of the divorce proceedings. I am not sure what that says about poetry, but the group laughed at hearing this gossip and added that perhaps Picasso just had a broken heart.

A collection of Picasso's poetry was published in *The Burial of the Count of Orgaz & Other Poems,* co-edited by Jerome Rothenberg and Pierre Joris. We shared samples of Picasso's poetry, including "Sky," which reads in part:

. . . sky sky sky sky sky sky sky sky sky violet violet sky sky sky violet violet violet sky sky sky violet violet violet sky sky sky . . .

We talked about how with the use of repeated words you could create poems with an element of Cubism. We felt that his poem "Her Great Thighs" blended well with *Les Demoiselles d'Avignon,* and Francesca and I performed the poem as a duet. Here is a small sample:

Her great thighs
Her breasts
Her hips
Her buttocks

. . .

Her nose
Her throat
Her tears

Another way to pair poetry and art is to use poems written in tribute to the artist. We turned to a section of Gertrude Stein's "A Completed Portrait of Picasso," with its circular repetitions. I had listened to recordings of Stein reading her poetry and had learned to mimic her tone and cadence. Taking on her voice, I led the group in a performance of a section of the poem using call and response. The participants enjoyed the playfulness of Stein's language, which always makes so much more sense to me when it is read aloud:

. . . If I told him would he like it. Would he like it if I told him.
Would he like it would Napoleon
would Napoleon would would he like it . . .

Sleeping Gypsy

We moved on to Rousseau's *Sleeping Gypsy.* With this painting I had found a description of a banquet that Picasso had thrown for Rousseau in 1908 and the poem "Ode to Rousseau," which was written for the occasion by the French poet Andre Salmon, who had stood on a bench at the party and recited the poem (http://www.bonjourparis.com/story/glory-years-henri-rousseau-1/).

We tapped into the group's creativity by asking them to imagine they were at the party. Meet Me at MoMA using the technique of "turn and talk," which encourages participants to engage each other in discussion around a painting. We used this technique with *Sleeping Gypsy*. Francesca talked about the artists' friendships and the Parisian salon and café scenes. We talked about Guillaume Apollinaire, a French poet, playwright, and novelist of the early twentieth century, and how he championed his artist friends in poems and essays. I quoted from the verse he wrote for Rousseau's gravestone. Then we engaged in the second art cheer of the day by holding up imaginary glasses of wine and toasting with Salmon's poem. Here is an excerpt:

. . . To honor you, for it is time to drink it
Crying all in chorus, Long Live! Long live Rousseau . . .

Starry Night

Having performed poems and discussed and focused on artwork for the past 30 minutes as a kind of warm-up and imagination primer, we then moved on to our last artwork and the one we would spend the next 30 to 45 minutes with: van Gogh's *Starry Night*.

In researching connections between van Gogh and poetry, I was greatly aided by the wonderful collection of his letters that can be found on the Vincent van Gogh Museum website (http://www.vangoghmuseum.nl/vgm/index.jsp). You are able to search his letters by term, to see the original letters, and to read them in various languages. They are also annotated with hypertext links, which proved invaluable.

I typed *poetry* into the search box and came up with 25 quotes from van Gogh in which he commented about how poetry inspired him and what place it had in his life.

The first thing I discovered was that van Gogh would take poems that he liked, copy them longhand, and then sew them into a collection for his brother, Theo. The thought of him making these little chapbooks is delightful. One of the poems he copied for Theo was Longfellow's "Afternoon in February," with its images of light and color. I printed out the poem with enlarged type to make it easier for the participants to read and during the tour had a volunteer from the group read it aloud:

The day is ending
The night descending
The marsh is frozen
The river dead.

Through clouds like ashes
The red sun flashes
On village windows
That glimmer red.

And through the meadows
Like fearful shadows
Slowly passes
a funeral train.

In a letter to Theo written from London in January 1874, van Gogh writes:

> Things are going well for me here, I have a wonderful home and it's a great pleasure for me to observe London and the English way of life and the English themselves, and I also have nature and art and poetry, and if that isn't enough, what is?

I was thrilled when I found another quote from van Gogh, in which he raves about one of America's most beloved poets, Walt Whitman. He wrote to his sister, Willemien van Gogh, in August 1888 from Arles in the south of France:

> Have you read Whitman's American poems yet? Theo should have them, and I really urge you to read them, first because they're really beautiful, and also, English people are talking about them a lot at the moment. He sees in the future, and even in the present, a world of health, of generous, frank carnal love—of friendship—of work, with the great starry firmament, something, in short, that one could only call God and eternity, put back in place above this world. They make you smile at first, they're so candid, and then they make you think, for the same reason.

This led me to an essay, "Whitman and van Gogh: Starry Nights and Other Similarities," which was written by Hope B. Werness, an academic researcher, and published in the 1985 *Walt Whitman Quarterly Review*. Werness quotes from a number of Whitman's poems, including "Song of Myself." In the article, she remarks on the similarities in the poet's and artist's philosophy and in seeing themselves as forging new art. Werness discusses how this is evident in Whitman's poems and van Gogh's painted visions of the night sky.

In December of 1888, van Gogh underwent his famous breakdown. Fearing for his sanity, he voluntarily committed himself to the asylum at Saint Rémy. It was during that stay in 1889 that he painted *Starry Night*, with its swirling images. Writing simply to Theo on June 18th, "At last, I have a landscape with olive trees, and also a new study of a starry sky."

As a group, we performed a section from "Song of Myself" using call and response:

Speeding through space, speeding through heaven and the stars,
Speeding amid the seven satellites and the broad ring,
   and the diameter of eighty thousand miles,
Speeding with tail'd meteors, throwing fire-balls like the rest,
Carrying the crescent child that carries its own full mother in its belly,
Storming, enjoying, planning, loving, cautioning,
Backing and filling, appearing and disappearing,
I tread day and night such roads. (Whitman, *Leaves of Grass,* pp. 64–65)

To end the tour, we shifted to creating our own poem inspired by *Starry Night*. I asked a series of questions around the painting, eliciting the group's thoughts on how the painting made them feel. We explored the images in the painting, focusing on the stars. I asked what stars might taste, smell, and sound like.

When I ask a group what they like best about Meet Me at MoMA, participants always mention how during these tours they feel like the museum is theirs. Standing as close to *Starry Night* as van Gogh did when he painted it, I felt the same.

To see a performance of the finished poem, go to the APP YouTube Channel at http://www.youtube.com/watch?v = iN-yJlt8hMA.

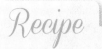
Recipe

VINCENT'S HONEST HUNGER

INGREDIENTS:

1 **museum** (A gallery will do if museums are scarce, or substitute using any artistic image.)
1 **work of art** (You know what you like!)
2 **hungry eyes** (or more)
2 **open minds** (or more)
1 **blank sheet of paper** (or more)
1 **writing utensil** (or more)

INSTRUCTIONS:

I like to take a few deep breaths and look at the artwork from a little way back, roughly 10 feet or so, then move in closer (or as close as the museum will allow). Spend time focusing on different areas of the artwork, then take a look at it overall. After you feel you have absorbed the artwork, you are ready to begin .

You may frame the questions in many ways:

Describe what you see in the artwork.

What about the colors in the artwork? Which do you see?

What do you like about the artwork?

What don't you like?

What feeling does it give you?

What does it make you think about?

These are just a few lines of questions. You may take this lesson in many interesting directions. Try using our old standby of exploring the artwork or elements of the artwork with your senses, as we did with van Gogh's *Starry Night*.

Write down the responses, which will become the lines of the poem. End by performing the newly created poem using the technique of call and response or read the poem to each other.

Stir gently and have fun!

CommuniTea
Creating an Event Around Sharing Tea

The cherry blossoms at the Brooklyn Botanical Garden were at peak pink bloom, or as the Japanese poet Matsudaira Sadanobu wrote, ". . . with branches so gentle, flowers so delicate in shape, and hues so simple that the total effect is perfect beyond belief."

I wandered into a room where the walls were draped with lovely oversized tea bags. They had been tinted by dipping them in tea, which created a wonderful patina of brown and gold. I was enchanted and then I realized that the tea bags were covered with writing, many of them poems. I knew I had to meet the artist, Michele Brody. She was chatting with people attending the exhibit. I introduced myself and learned that she called this work, "Reflections in Tea." She had asked the people attending the exhibit to write their own stories about tea. It was a delightful way to encourage people to participate in the art experience.

I told Michele about my work with the Alzheimer's Poetry Project and we began to talk about ways to collaborate. I invited her to attend a workshop at New York Memory Center. She brought in tins of different scented teas and I collected a group of poems about tea, other beverages, and drinking. We passed around the teas and read the poems. We then created our own poem about tea.

This led us to invite Michele to be a guest artist at one of our Memory Arts Café events. Memory Arts Café is a series of free art events for people living with Alzheimer's disease, their caregivers, and the general public and is co-produced by New York Memory Center and the APP. The series includes light refreshments and the opportunity to chat with the guest artists. In general, people really love sharing conversation and poetry over tea.

APP created an elaborate event entitled "CommuniTea with Poetry" when Michele had a residency with the Hudson Guild at the Fulton Center in Manhattan. As many of the people who attend the Fulton Center speak Spanish, we did the program in English and Spanish. Again we used poems about tea, including many haiku by the Japanese poet Kobayashi Issa. We asked the Spanish-speaking participants to help translate the poems. This allowed them to be the experts and was great fun for us all.

With CommuniTea, the serving of the tea became an integral part of the event. Michele brought in a teakettle that whistled when the water was boiling. She also brought in cookies. One of the groups at Fulton Center had been working on ceramics, so they added handmade teacups that were delightful to hold and look at.

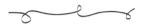

FOR OUR ELDERS WITH MEMORY LOSS
FABU

Some call you seniors
I call you wise elders
Living long and learning much.

You should be honored
Your grey hair a symbol
Of victory and authority in life.

When your memory flees or hides
And every face seem strange
Remember the other signs of love.

The gentle touch, the kind voice
The spirit that welcomes you
Just as you are.

Reassure yourselves
That you know how love feels
For it will chase the fear of forgetting
away.

MICHELE BRODY'S WORLD-CHAMPION POT OF TEA POEMS

INGREDIENTS:

1 generous scoop of tea
  (We used black teas from China, but please use your favorite.)
1 whistling teapot
2 teacups (or more)
2 empty minds (or more)
2 welcoming spirits (or more)

INSTRUCTIONS:

In loose order, here are steps for conducting a CommuniTea program:

Participants enter and are greeted and seated.

Each group member selects a teacup.

Opening poem is read. (We used my poem, "Tea" [see below].)

Person leading the program describes what will happen during the event.

Participants sniff both the brewed and loose teas.

Tea is poured. (We made a big deal of the pouring by adding flourishes.)

Conversation ensues. (About the tea, but also just chatting.)

Poems are performed using call and response.

Group poem is created. (We asked open-ended questions about tea and sharing beverages.)

Participants are invited to perform the group poem.

Conversation continues and eventually good-byes are said. (People really lingered and did not want to leave.)

Tips on Tea Poem Selection:

We use many haiku by the Japanese poet Kobayashi Issa. He eventually took the pen name Issa, which means "cup of tea," or, according to poet

continued

Robert Hass, "a single bubble in steeping tea." These are easy to find on-line. An especially good resource for Issa's haiku is on David Lanoue web-site, The Hakiu Guy (http://haikuguy.com/issa/). Lanoue has translated Issa's work into many books, including *Cup of Tea Poems*.

Tea Poems

We used the following poems at the CommuniTea event to give the spirit of sharing beverages, including a poem of mine, which we used as the introduction to the event.

A Drinking Song
WILLIAM BUTLER YEATS

Wine comes in at the mouth
And love comes in at the eye;
That's all we know for truth
Before we grow old and die.
I lift the glass to my mouth,
I look at you, and I sigh.

Song to Celia
BEN JONSON

(Opening lines)

Drink to me only with thine eyes,
And I will pledge with mine;
Or leave a kiss but in the cup,
And I'll not look for wine.

A Young Lady of Lynn
ANONYMOUS

There was a young lady of Lynn,
Who was so uncommonly thin
That when she essayed
To drink lemonade
She slipped through the straw and fell in.

continued

Tea

GARY GLAZNER

Steam is the first sip,
touching the air with taste.
Scent is the second sip,
the tang of union.

Too hot—
hint of purity, lips recoil.
Now the waiting,
place hands on the edge of vessel.
Listen for cooling.

No one knows where the drink comes from,
it shows up in the kitchen a guest.
Be a good host: ask the kettle why it sings.

Caress the handle with flesh.
Open your mouth to its mouth.
Inhale the last drop of honey.
What pleasure the empty cup knows.

You work with what you are given,
the red clay of grief,
the black clay of stubbornness going on after.
Clay that tastes of care or carelessness,
clay that smells of the bottoms of rivers or dust.

FROM "REBUS," BY JANE HIRSHFIELD

Clay as Poetry

One of the most creative art projects the Alzheimer's Poetry Project has been involved in is through our Minnesota chapter. Poets Zoë Bird and Rachel Moritz worked with clay artist Angie Renee as part of the Wilder Foundation's Adult Day Health program in Minneapolis to create sculptures of poetry and clay.

Zoë Bird and Rachel Moritz Describe the Clay and Poetry Workshop

The project began with poetry and ended with the clay workshops. As teaching artists, our first step was to brainstorm the kinds of poems and clay creations we thought would work best and fully engage participants. Our overall goal was to create something beautiful, tangible, durable, and unique that could live in the outdoor garden space at Wilder Adult Day Health and marry the two art forms of poetry and clay. In a previous year, Wilder had used sidewalk chalk and simple painted signs for displaying our garden poems, but these had neither the durability nor the beauty of something made from clay.

After deciding on themes for the garden projects—butterflies and vegetables—we led poetry classes with two groups at Wilder: individuals in the Day Room (Wilder's general day program), and those in the Great Room (the memory-loss group). Day Room participants wrote about butterflies, and Great Room participants worked on a poem about vegetable gardens.

We sent both poems to Angie Renee, who gave the clay process some thought. Originally, we had hoped to match individual poetic lines to each participant, who could then work on a unique clay tile or sculpture to accompany his or her words. However, this proved too logistically complicated, as individuals come on different days and to different classes

---

at Wilder Adult Day Health. In the end, Angie stamped the words of the poems into the clay tiles without attributing individual lines.

Angie conducted two clay workshops, one to complete the Butterfly Garden tiles and one for the Vegetable Garden. Participants worked either on individual vegetable tiles or as a group on the butterfly tiles. We ended both clay sessions with a call-and-response reading of the poems. After the clay tiles had been fired and finished, Angie completed final assembly installation in the garden space.

Model Poems Used in the Sessions

For the Butterfly Garden poem, we used the following model poems:

W. B. Yeats's "A110" (from *The Collected Works of W. B. Yeats, Volume I: The Poems, Second Edition*):

To Garret or Cellar a wheel I send,
But every butterfly to a friend.

"Caterpillars," by Brod Bagert

"The Search for Lost Lives," by James Tate

The following are other examples of poems for garden sessions:

"This Compost," by Walt Whitman (excerpt from)

"Vegetable-Life," by Ned O'Gorman (excerpt from)

"My Garden with Walls," by William Brooks

"How to Get a Garden," by Andrew Roberts, age 4, from the anthology *For Kids, By Kids*

The two garden creations capture in physical form the poetry we do every week with participants at Wilder Adult Day Health, and people can look at them again and again. This was a perfect collaboration, both of artistic medium and of teaching artists.

Angie Renee's Clay as Poetry Tips

- Have fun, and remind the folks not to be too critical of themselves.

- Tell them they can do it, even if they have never worked with clay before.

- Show each person how to do things simply, like roll a coil between their hands. When you break things down, it often moves them past their blocks.

ANGIE RENNE'S STRAIGHT-UP RECIPE FOR A WALKING GARDEN POEM

INGREDIENTS:

2 poets (Zoë Bird and Rachel Moritz)
1 clay artist (Angie Renne)
1 group poem

Add in:
1 classroom with 12 willing artists
12 forks
12 wooden stick tools
12 paint brushes

Placed on:
12 red trays lined with newspaper
12 tiles of clay (include extra clay for all)

Most important addition:
12 creative minds
24 hands to create with

Ending with:
15 smiles

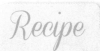

ZOË'S BUTTERFLY POETRY SESSION
(Time needed: 1 or 2 hours of prep time; 1-hour session)

INGREDIENTS:

1 room full of poets

1 encyclopedia of butterflies or other butterfly book;
butterfly props and images (postcards and puppets are fun)

2 or 3 model poems. Some successful examples:

- W.B. Yeats's A110:
  "To a Garret or Cellar a wheel I send, But every butterfly to a friend."
- James Tate's "The Search for Lost Lives"
- Brenda Cardenas's "Zacuanpapalotls"

1 easel with large notepad and markers

Optional:

several chrysalises, which will eventually become Monarch butterflies

Monarch butterfly in a jar, found and sent by a friend with a
fortune reading: "An unknown person will give you a diamond
larger than the size of an egg."

continued

INSTRUCTIONS:

- Introduce everyone and greet everyone by name. Express how happy you are to see them. Check in: "How's everybody doing?"

- Stretch. Move. Maybe bat a balloon around for a little while checking in. Bring out book, images, and props and pass them around.

- Recite a butterfly poem. Teaching artist may recite first, and then invite the group to join in using call and response.

- Use the poem to open a dialogue about butterflies. Get ready with the markers and start writing down lines. They'll be shared before you start deliberately gathering for the group poem.

- Use more model poems as needed, to keep the conversation going.

- Use open-ended questions (questions without a single right answer) to gather more lines for the group poem (e.g., "How do butterflies know how to be butterflies?" "How do you feel when you see a butterfly?" "What is transformation?")

- Recite the group poem together using call and response.

- If lacking a title for the group poem, cast about for one.

- Congratulate all of the poets on making a wonderful poem!

- Take home and type up the poem. Distribute and post, where possible.

- Collaborate with other artists to extend the life of the poem and transform it further—butterfly-like—by using it as the inspiration for works of art in other media (by the participating poets and others).

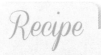
Recipe

RACHEL'S EVERYTHING GARDEN POETRY SESSION
(Time needed: 1 hour of prep time; 1-hour session; half-hour to type poem)

INGREDIENTS:

A sunny, summer day is best

Comfortable outdoor seating (benches, chairs). If there is a garden or
growing flowers nearby, all the better.

Poetry participants (anywhere from 4–12). It helps if they are wearing
hats to shield from the sun.

Vegetable props to include: ripe tomato, zucchini, cucumber, red
onion, garlic, radish, and some fragrant herbs (basil, sage, parsley)

1 or 2 model poems. Some successful examples:

- "Digging Potatoes, Sebago, Maine," by Amy E. King (This is a
  long poem. I suggest the second half only.)
- "Cauliflower," by Gladys Wellington (This is a great poem to use for
  a conversation about family, siblings, and parents; vegetables are merely
  metaphors.)
- "Parsley," Jeannette Ferrary (This poem helps introduce some humor;
  gotta have parsley in hand for this one!)

1 or 2 interesting quotes about vegetables (e.g., "Shall I not have intel-
ligence with the earth? Am I not partly leaves and vegetable mould myself.
[Henry David Thoreau]).

1 easel with large notepad and markers

continued

INSTRUCTIONS:

Introduce everyone and ask how they are doing. "Are you comfortable?" "Too hot?" "Too cold?" Admire the garden and the outdoor space in which you are sitting. Talk about summertime and all its glories.

Pass around vegetables one by one, asking participants to feel free to touch and smell them, as well as taste the herbs. Ask if they can guess the herb variety. Ask if anyone is gardening at home or has in the past. What are people growing? What have they grown in the past? As vegetables go around the circle, chat about favorites or least favorites.

Recite a garden poem. Teaching artist may read the full poem first and then invite participants to recite it line-by-line for the second reading.

Use the poem to open a dialogue about gardens, with the following questions as prompts: "What would you plant in your garden?" (suggested poem: "Digging up Potatoes, Sebago, Maine"); "If you were a vegetable, which one would you like to be?" (suggested poems: "Cauliflower" or "Parsley").

Begin to write down responses on the easel notepad, inviting participants to recite the lines with you as they are spoken. Recite more model poems as needed, to keep the conversation going.

Recite the group poem together using call and response.

Ask for consensus on a title.

Thank everyone for their artistry and creativity.

Ask if anyone would like to take a vegetable home with them!

Type up the poem and give copies to participants the next time you see them.

Fabiana's GoldMind

Fabiana Glazer is the dynamic founder and Director of GoldMind Arts and Aging, an organization dedicated to improving quality of life through the creative experience. Fabiana is herself a successful painter whose work can be found in numerous private collections in the United States and Europe. I met Fabiana at the Museum of Modern Art (MoMA) Leadership Exchange in 2013. She is the daughter of Robin Glazer, who runs the Creative Center in the Lower East Side in New York. As our last names have a very similar spelling, people have commented on how much they enjoyed meeting my daughter and, by the way, when did Robin and I break up? So I am really happy to be able to include here my "art" daughter "Fabi" and her amazing recipes combing poetry, art viewing, and art making. Her work is truly a GoldMind!

(Gary) How did you start using art with elders?

(Fabiana) I started working with elders as many of us in the field did—from personal experience. My grandmother passed away from complications of dementia, and she suffered very much towards the end of her life. In the limited time I had to work with her, creating art in the day center she attended, I realized the importance and power of using art with older adults living with memory disorder.

(Gary) Describe the workshops you hold at University of Chicago Medicine.

(Fabiana) My work at University of Chicago Medicine through the Memory Center is an innovative and joyous program. The patients are all referred to the program by their neurologist, which sends a powerful message about the importance of art in dementia care. The participants are individuals living with memory disorders and their caregivers. The staff of the facility, which is also the primary care center for the participants, are very enthusiastic about the program and frequently drop in and do art over lunch, too.

This weekly class is based on methods from MoMA's Alzheimer's Project, the Alzheimer's Poetry Project, and Mark Morris Dance Group for PD [Parkinson's disease], along with techniques I have developed at GoldMind Arts. We use visual art, poetry, movement, music, and even flavor to stimulate and engage participants.

Evaluations indicate many benefits, including improving caregiver/care staff/patient relationships, decreasing depression, increased activity outside of class, increased verbalization, and a strong desire to continue attending the program!

(Gary) What is your greatest challenge?

(Fabiana) My greatest challenge is the very first step—getting new participants in the door. Depression, inactivity, and fear are unpleasant but common side effects of dementia, and they can present a real challenge. Once that individual is in the room, they are almost always drawn towards the art making and fully engage with the group. It is natural and normal for a human being to learn, create, and forge relationships. I have learned that a 5-minute conversation with a new potential participant can be enough to break the first-time barrier. It takes a smile and a hand to get started sometimes!

(Gary) Anything else you care to add?

(Fabiana) I love this work. Throughout my career as a teaching artist, I have worked with almost every age group and special populations. My work with people living with dementia is by far the most rewarding, challenging, and needed. Thanks to the stigmas towards aging and chronic illness in general, this group is sorely lacking resources. These art programs have an enormous impact, and I feel incredibly proud to be working in this field.

MS. FABI'S COLOR TALKS

INGREDIENTS:

1 poem ("Colors, Colors, Colors," by Peter S. Quinn)

1 observed art (e.g., Rothko and Albers, or substitute almost any works by these artists)

1 large number of paint color sample cards of countless colors from a large box home improvement store

1 passel of glue sticks

INSTRUCTIONS:

After introductions, play with the poem and talk about the paintings, which usually leads to the relationship of color, the subjectivity, and the interpretation. The participants are always able to share from their personal experiences and create common memories and meaning.

Spread the large number of paint color sample cards of countless colors over a whole table. Encourage the participants to "talk in color," using the various colors to express themselves instead of words. As the group questions such as "What are you like in the morning?" "What does the night look like?" and "What do you wish for?" Finally, ask the participants to describe themselves and each other in color.

Mount the color sample cards to card stock with glue sticks.

Bonus:

The participants can bring home the work they created at the end of class.

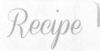

BIRDS ON A WIRE

INGREDIENTS:

1 Poem ("I Know Why The Caged Bird Sings," by Maya Angelou)
1 observed art (Dove of Peace, by Picasso)
1 ball of twine
1 window frame
1 stack of colorful card stock
15 pounds of feathers (or less)
1 bag of Mardi Gras beads
1 passel of glue sticks
1 flock of scissors

INSTRUCTIONS:

After introductions, playing with the poem, and talking about the drawing, engage the group in a discussion of birds as a symbol and the meanings of freedom.

The participants are always able to share from their personal experiences and create common memories and meaning.

After mounting a few pieces of twine inside the window frame of the classroom, ask each member of the class to create a bird from colorful card stock and decorate them with feathers, paper, etc.

Hang the birds on the twine, as if looking out the window, with small paper clips. The art remains in the space as an installation, beautifying the space!

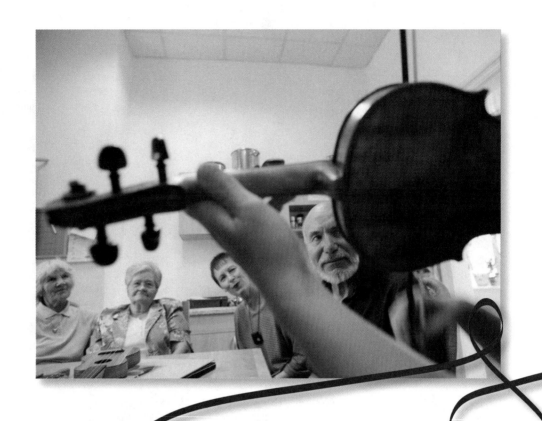

Five
MUSIC

Life is one long jubilee.
—IRA GERSHWIN

Life is a lot like jazz ... it's best when you improvise.
—GEORGE GERSHWIN

Poem and Song Medley

The Alzheimer's Poetry Project has had a lot of fun in its poetry sessions creating performances by alternating saying the lines of a poem with singing the lyrics of a song. This exercise can be done with a group of family and friends or one-on-one with your loved one. The technique can lend itself to many poems and songs.

Many of the songs I have chosen happen to be favorites of some of the people I work with at the New York Memory Center. I choose the poems to accompany the songs partially based on words or themes that link the song and poem and partially because they are favorite poems of mine. Talking with your family and friends about favorite songs to sing and thinking of what poems might go with the songs is part of the pleasure of creating a poem and song medley.

Example One

In this first example we will mix the last stanza of the "Owl and the Pussy Cat," by Edward Lear, with the opening lines to "Fly Me to the Moon," by Bert Howard. I like the Frank Sinatra version of the song, but there are many other recordings of the song, including wonderful versions by Peggy Lee, Tony Bennett, Diana Krall, and Nat King Cole. If you are not familiar with the song, please listen to one the recordings. Please also find and print the lyrics to "Fly Me to the Moon" via the Internet.

Step 1. Start by reciting the last stanza of the poem. You can clap along to the rhythm of the poem. Repeat three to four times to build up enthusiasm:

And hand in hand, on the edge of the sand,
They danced by the light of the moon,
The moon,
The moon,
They danced by the light of the moon.

Step 2. When you finish the stanza, sing the first verse of "Fly Me to the Moon."

Fly me to the moon
Let me play among the stars
Let me see what spring is like
On Jupiter and Mars
In other words, hold my hand
In other words, baby, kiss me

Step 3. When you get to the line, "In other words, baby, kiss me," go back into the poem chanting:

And hand in hand, on the edge of the sand,
They danced by the light of the moon,
The moon,
The moon,
They danced by the light of the moon.

Step 4. Alternate between the poem and song until finished.

Example Two

In the second example, we will mix up "America the Beautiful," by Katharine Lee Bates and Samuel A. Ward, with the Emma Lazarus poem "New Colossus," which celebrates the Statue of Liberty.

Step 1. Sing the first verse of "America the Beautiful":

O beautiful for spacious skies,
For amber waves of grain,
For purple mountain majesties
Above the fruited plain!
America! America!
God shed His grace on thee,
And crown thy good with brotherhood
From sea to shining sea!

Step 2. Say the following iconic lines from "New Colossus." Experiment with repeating the lines two or three times before going back into the song:

". . . Give me your tired, your poor, your huddled masses yearning to breathe free . . ."

Step 3. Alternate between the poem and song until finished.

Below are some other poem–song medley possibilities:

"Casey at the Bat" paired with "Take Me Out to the Ballgame"

"Twas the Night before Christmas" paired with "Silent Night" 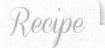 and/or "Jingle Bells"

"Fog" (Carl Sandberg) paired with "I Left My Heart in San Francisco"

"Pledge of Allegiance" paired with "This Land Is Your Land"

Recipe

GARY'S GRILLED POEM AND SONG MEDLEY

INGREDIENTS:

1 song (day old is fine)
1 poem (musty is best)
1 chorus of fearless motor mouths
1 bunch of ears
1 bucket (to carry tune)

INSTRUCTIONS:

Alternate between the song and poem. How much of each? You've just got to feel it out. Sing your heart out! Do not worry if your tune-carrying bucket leaks. When you get to the poem, go all gospel, shouting and praising and waving your hands. When you switch back to the song, stomp your feet or alternatively whisper. You will know how and when to alternate depending on the song and the mood you are trying to create. This should feel like a revival or a wake. Let the sunshine in, throw open the windows. If this recipe is done right, the neighbors may remark, "What in blue blazes is going on over there?" Peaking their heads in to take a look, they might be swept up in the goings on and join in: a big ole singing, marching, happy, happy poetry parade!

Blues Poetry Workshop

Zoë growled in her best blues voice "I am the 'Lemon Wolf of the Blues.'" Rachel exclaimed she was the "Tiny Princess of the Blues." Zoë told the group Bessie Smith was known as the "Empress of the Blues." Then they encouraged the group to give themselves blues names.

The blues poetry workshop idea is based on a session led by Zoë Bird and Rachel Moritz of Wilder Foundation's Adult Day Health in Minneapolis, Minnesota. Zoë introduced Bessie Smith to the group and explained that blues was a style of music created by African-Americans in the southern United States. While blues often expresses sadness, the music is not always sad. In fact, you can dance to some blues tunes.

Outside of blues royalty, such as B. B. King (the "The King of the Blues"), there are blues musicians and bands whose names are based on how fast you are, such as Lightnin' Hopkins, as well as lots of size monikers, such as Little Walter and Big Bill Broonzy. Your name could be where you come from (Mississippi John Hurt), a reference to your body (Peg Leg Howell), a food preference (Barbecue Bob), or your ability to eat anything (Lead Belly). You get the idea—encourage the group to have fun with choosing their names!

Zoë and Rachel then played a YouTube video of Bessie Smith singing "Backwater Blues." They also showed the group a well-known photo of Smith by Carl Van Vechten, so they could see what she looked like as well as hear her singing. Then Zoë led the group in a call-and-response rendition of "Backwater Blues."

After the wonderful opening mix of performance, listening, and joy and humor in creating blues names, Zoë and Rachel moved on to creating a poem with the group. Rachel asked the group to finish the line, "I woke up in the morning . . . ," and Zoë wrote down the responses, which became the lines of the poem. Rachel moved around the room, kneeling down to be close to each person as he or she gave a response. This helped the group members to focus and gave the shy ones a chance to whisper their responses in her ear. The group created the poem that follows.

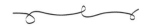

SUPER-GREAT BLUES, FROM ALL OF US
THE WILDER ADULT DAY HEALTH POETS FROM THE DAY AND GREAT ROOMS

I'm the tiny princess of the blues,
I'm the wiggly guy of the blues!
I can stick with the blues.
I'm the keeper of the blues.
The Ella Fitzgerald of the blues.
The Kennedy of the blues!
I'm the smiling face of the blues.
I cry with the blues.
I think I'm Fonzie of the blues—
two thumbs up!
I play with the blues,
blues in my soul,
blues in my Kennedy.

I woke up this morning,
started on my way—
I woke up this morning
and I was so cold
I had to put on a sweater.
I woke up this morning,
I put a bowl on my head
and gave myself a haircut!
I woke up this morning
and I put on a sweater, too—
I can't find my earrings
and I can't find my other shoe.

I woke up this morning
and I was anxious to get over here!
Conductor of the blues,
I can't find my snowshoes.
I'd sing the blue velvet blues,
and I'd be the lemon wolf of the blues—
I said that for a reason!

I'm the ringleader of the blues.
I've got the blues in my heart
and I don't know where to start.

You already asked me the first time,
and this time should be the last.
Don't ask me a second time,
'cause I can't remember!
What did I tell you—
I've got the you-never-listen-to-me blues.

I've got the cool blues.
I'm teaching the children the blues
in my red shoes.
The blue-sky blues
go play in the puddles.

I woke up this morning,
had my strong coffee
with a little cream.
I woke up this morning,
had my tea
with a little cream.
The kind I like.
Heinz 57,
put 'em all together,
make a brew
the witches in Salem would like.
That's not Oregon,
that's Massachusetts—
make no mistake!

I woke up this morning
and I went right over to play the piano,
I was so blue—
because I have to go to the dentist today.
Sounds like the blues
are gonna go on forever,
till the end of time.

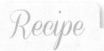 *Recipe*

WORLD CHAMPION RECIPE FOR THE BLUES

INGREDIENTS:

1 or more blues song recording
1 or more blues song lyrics
1 tear in your heart and a bad man or woman (your preference) on your mind

PERFORMANCE TIPS:

Listen to a song to get you in the mood. If you are feeling it, maybe sing along. Then perform the lyrics with the group using call and response. Talk about how the blues are not always sad, how blues music was often dance music, and how the blues had a baby and named it Rock 'n' Roll. Give examples of blues names and have everyone choose a blues name. Next, take a typical blues lyrics and ask the group to finish the thoughts:

I woke up in the morning and _____
I'm going down that river, I'm going _____
Baby, please don't go, oh, baby, please don't go. Baby, please don't go down to _____

For these next lyrics, encourage the group to think of wild, creative places for Baby to not go to:

Don't go to the moon
Don't go to bottom of the ocean
Don't go back in time
Don't go into the mouth of a lion

And then switch it up to give example of where baby should go:

Please go into my arms
Please go to church
Please go to the store and buy me some ice cream

Write down the responses and perform the blues poem using call and response, perhaps singing some of the lines in your best Howlin' Wolf, Muddy Waters, or Bessie Smith blues voice.

continued

All the Blues in the World
GARY GLAZNER

Head down to the crossroads
Pushing your little red rooster
In your little red wheelbarrow
So much depends upon a
spoonful of coffee or a spoonful of tea
A Wang Dang Doodle and a little red poodle
Your Hoochie Coochie pooch
Yes, a hellhound on your trail
Dusting your broom
All your love in vain
You got the Walking Blues
You got the Empty Bed Blues
And by the time you get to Sweet Home Chicago
You need a little sugar in you bowl,
You need a little hot dog, on you roll
I'm gonna buy you a diamond ring
And if that diamond ring don't sing
Bop bopa-a-lu a whop bam boo
I got a recipe for the blues for you.
Um hmmm that's right yeah!
I got a recipe for the blues for you.
Ha! Lilin! Lidilin! Eh!
Hooooo YEAH!
So sad so very, very sad . . .

Jazz and Poetry
A Technique to Build Performance Skills

With Jazz music blazing, I was shouting poetry at Chrysler Headquarters in Detroit. The auto industry team was trying to be cool and snap their fingers to the beat, but part of the celebratory spread being served was chicken wings, so many of their fingers were too greasy to snap.

My absolute dream job, or as they say in the jazz world "dream gig," was to tour with a jazz band. It came true when Pontiac wanted to promote its new car the Vibe by hiring the jazz band Vibes to tour around the country playing gigs and making the car hip and cool to young people. A marketing genius decided that the perfect accessory to the jazz band would be a poet. The event in Detroit was to honor the team that had worked on the Vibe.

They called it the Beat Tour, harkening back to the beatniks and beat poets of the 1950s. Pontiac made poetry magnets to attach to the car, so when we parked in front of a venue people could create poems by rearranging the words. The poetry magnets stayed on the car really well until we hit 60 miles an hour, at which time they began to fly off the sides. We always knew when we hit 60 by the dirty looks the other drivers gave us.

We did 25 performances across the country, starting in New York and ending in Los Angeles. The band was a fantastic trio, with Bill Ware on vibraphone, Bard Jones on bass, and E. J. Rodriguez on drums. They had worked as the rhythm section for the Jazz Passengers, whose lead singer was Deborah Harry of Blondie fame. They had played with many of the leading jazz musicians, and Ware had played with Steely Dan and the BBC Orchestra.

In performing with Vibes, I had a chance to try out many ideas I had on combining poetry with music. Try out the recipe that follows.

COOKING WITH CHARLIE PARKER SAUCE

INGREDIENTS:

1 or more blues song recording
1 or more blues song lyrics
1 tear in your heart and a bad man or woman (your preference)
on your mind

INSTRUCTIONS:

Try reading the poem over the jazz recording. Match the emotion in your voice to the emotion of the music. Match the speed of your recitation to the tempo of the music. Does the music have a certain color or feel? Try to create that with your voice. Have fun and try different voices, tones, and colors to see what works and what does not.

After you have practiced with a recording, perhaps you have a friend who plays an instrument and you can jam with. Try out the ideas you have worked on with the recording with a live musician. Have a blast!

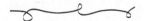

RECIPE FOR A POTION TO MAKE SOMEONE DISAPPEAR (*excerpt*)
MICHELLE OTERO AND THE POETS OF NORTH VALLEY SHARE YOUR CARE

Start with something that's sharp.

How about 12 bat wings
to make them fly away?

Add some disappearing liquid,
a cup per person.

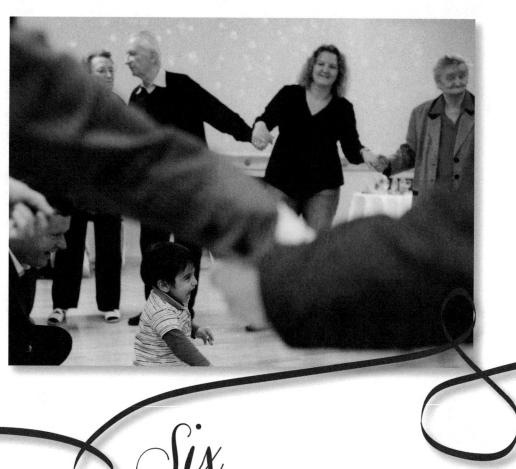

Six
MOVEMENT

Square Dancing to Poetry

When I was in first grade, I won a twist contest. What little I remember of the experience is that as the winner, the teacher brought me to other classrooms to demonstrate my dance prowess and there was a lot of pointing and shouting as I dipped all the way to the floor, my little body twisting. That's how proud the teacher was that I was her student.

It was 1964, and the big hit on the radio was "I Want to Hold Your Hand," by the Beatles. On the way home from school the bus driver sang the song and everyone joined in with him. I have no recollection of how I learned to dance the twist, but I do have a very strong memory of sneaking at night with the other kids behind the apartment building where we all lived to catch fireflies, while the parents sat on the tiny apartment lawns in folding lawn chairs and ordered pizza for delivery just after midnight to circumvent

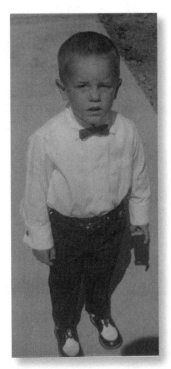

the Catholic's "meatless Fridays." As the parents counted the minutes to pizza nirvana, we would tire of chasing fireflies and catching them in jars and began dancing instead.

We called our dance the jelly, jelly cha, cha, cha. We would pair up boy and girl and turn our backs to each other, rubbing our bottoms together as we chanted: jelly, jelly cha, cha, cha, jelly, jelly cha, cha, cha!

Those late night dance sessions are what must have propelled me to win the twist contest in first grade. Or perhaps it was watching Fred Flintstone do a parody of the twist called "the twitch." Like millions of others, I had watched the Beatles on the Ed Sullivan show sing "Twist and Shout," so twisting was in the air.

This sense of playfulness I embodied at an early age still affects the energy I like to bring to my poetry sessions. While working in an assisted living or adult day center, a little humor and playfulness can really change the tone of a session and lift everyone's spirit. It also helps people get over their fear of poetry as being hard to understand or too stuffy.

Are you afraid of poetry? Did a teacher make you memorize a poem and then have you stand in front of the class and recite it, knees knocking and palms sweating while your classmates mocked your recitation? Most people hear poetry and run for the door. Try instead to remember that poetry can be funny and also fun to dance to. Humor is your friend and your secret weapon. Will you dance with me?

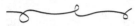

ALZPOETRY BREIDENBACK
LARS RUPPLE

I want to crumble
Whip cream
Leave myself behind
Clack with plates
Climb in the space between the tines of a dinner fork
Eat with my hands
Eat with my legs
Dance with my tongue
My teeth are lions
And the teeth of those lions
Are lions too
Lingering in the prairie
On a silent hunt
Their preys are gazelles made of dough
Crispy bite-sized sixteenth
Baked by the sun
Crispy and old?
I want to crumble

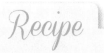

OPEN-FACED CHA CHA CHA JELLY JELLY

INGREDIENTS:

1 rhythmic poem
4 or more clapping hands
4 or more dancing feet

INSTRUCTIONS:

For this activity we will use the last two lines of "Daffodils," by Wordsworth. Start by reciting three times and use call and response to engage the group:

And then my heart with pleasure fills
And dances with the daffodils

When it feels right, kick it up a notch by clapping along with the rhythm of the poem, keeping the chant going. Again, you are going by feeling here, so as the energy builds, repeat it another four or so times.

And then my heart with pleasure fills
And dances with the daffodils.

At this point in the session, I reach my hand out to someone on staff and, while still chanting the poem, I start to *"dosido,"* hooking arm-in-arm and spinning around with the person in a square dance. Now the poem is really cooking and I start to switch up the last line. First with this variation:

And then my heart with pleasure fills
And dances with the dollar bills.

Then shifting to:

And then my heart with pleasure fills
And dances with the buffalo bills.

I alternate this technique to bring in humor and movement by holding the participant's hands and moving them to the rhythm of the poem. I typically end the dance by asking the person, "May I ask you a question, please? When you woke up this morning, did you think you would be square dancing to poetry?"

Poetry as Exercise

We were double-booked. The physical therapist and I had both been scheduled to lead a workshop at 10:30 a.m. We looked at each other and I asked, "Do you want to work together?" She said, "Yes." I proposed that she help the group create movements to the lines of a poem.

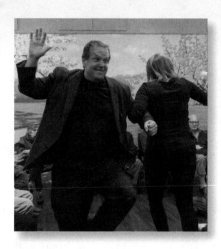

I chose "The Eagle," by Alfred, Lord Tennyson, and as I recited the lines, Tara helped the group respond to the words with simple movements. Here are the lines of the poem with descriptions of the movements.

The Eagle
(As you say the title, spread your arms out and move them like wings.)

He clasps the crag with crooked hands;
(Fingers take on the shape of a claw and dip down to grab a rock.)
Close to the sun in lonely lands.
(Arms up in a circle to indicate the sun.)
Below the azure world he stands.
(Hold arms in the circle.)
The wrinkled sea beneath him crawls;
(Hands forward making a waving motion.)
He watches from his mountain walls,
(Hand to forehead as lookout and to shade eyes from the sun.)
And like a thunderbolt
(Right arm extended up full length and to the right.)
he falls.
(Arm goes down and across body.)

Optional: Make an explosion sound as "thunderbolt" hits the water and follow the explosion sound by making a loud eagle cry while at the same time placing your hands cupped to your mouth to amplify the cry. If you are not sure what an eagle sounds like, try a rooster crow.

Once when I engaged a group in this activity, as I finished reciting the poem and the thunderbolt crashed into the water, a gentleman spread his arms out to the side in the universal baseball umpire gesture and shouted, "Safe!"

(Go to the following link to watch a performance of the poem with accompanying movement: http://www.youtube.com/watch?v = aC3ttkgpXSI)

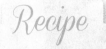

GARY'S FEEL THE BURN POETRY PARTY

> **INGREDIENTS:**
>
> 1 bunch of bodies
> 1 rhythmic, high-energy poem (or more, as needed)
> 1 peck of funky, good-time tunes

INSTRUCTIONS:

Put the tunes on just high enough to really feel the beat but not drown out your voice. Pick a movement (it does not have to be anything complicated), or ask the group what movement they want to do. Here are a few examples:

- Move your feet to the beat, alternating left and right.

- Thrust your arms out, alternating left and right like you are throwing punches.

- Raise your palms up to the sky, also known as "raising the roof."

You get the idea. Say the poem as you do the movements, matching the rhythm and tempo of the beat or pulse of the music. Then say the poem with the group using call and response. Repeat until you feel the burn!

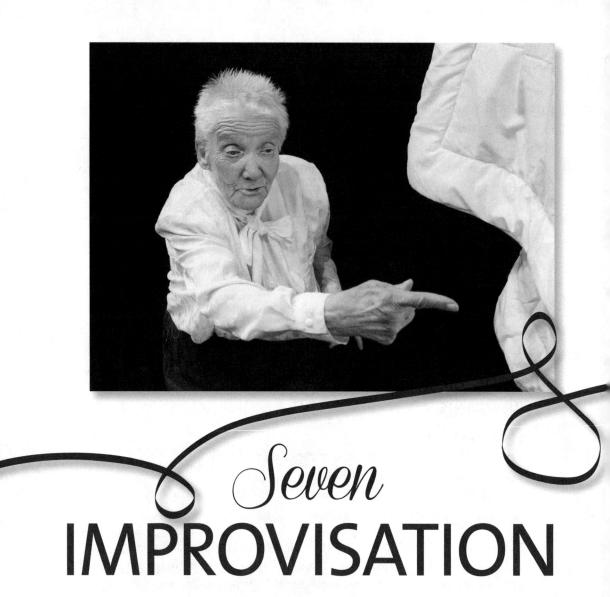

Seven
IMPROVISATION

Yes, and
Improvisation as a Communication Tool

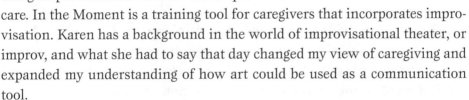

I felt like a giant light bulb had lit up over my head. I was listening to Karen Stobbe, founder of In the Moment, give a talk in 2005 at the Alzheimer's Foundation of America Conference in Dallas on using improvisational theater techniques in dementia care. In the Moment is a training tool for caregivers that incorporates improvisation. Karen has a background in the world of improvisational theater, or improv, and what she had to say that day changed my view of caregiving and expanded my understanding of how art could be used as a communication tool.

One lesson I learned from her was the concept of "Yes, and . . . " Stobbe says, "There is no more important rule in improvisation." The idea is that you "accept any offer made by another and that accepting helps move the action forward with additional information or action. But beyond that, it is also an important statement when fostering a positive attitude." This concept is central to all types of improv, including comedy. My guess is saying "yes, and" is central as well to the way jazz musicians improvise with each other.

In her speech to Harvard's graduating class of 2011, comedienne Amy Pohler shared her own "yes, and" advice:

> I moved to Chicago in the early 1990s and I studied improvisation there. I learned some rules that I try to apply still today: Listen. Say yes. Live in the moment. Even when it's uncomfortable, even when you are scared, saying yes helps you break through the barriers that hold you back in life. Saying yes will teach you, over and over again, that you are not the best judge of your capabilities. Saying yes opens doors that you have no idea even exist right now. So, SAY YES!

One technique that Stobbe uses to connect "Yes, and" to the world of Alzheimer's is by using it as a way to respond to the statement of "I want to go home." For example, if a person is saying "I want to go home," a typical answer might be "You are home," or "You can't go home; they sold your house," or "This is your home." If a person is genuinely requesting to go home, for whatever reason, you may make them more frustrated by not really listening and responding in a positive manner.

With "Yes, and" you can acknowledge someone who tells you he or she wants to go home by responding:

"Yes, and tell me about your home."

"Yes, and let's grab a jacket, it is a little chilly outside."

"Yes, and I could use your help right now."

Stobbe also points out that saying "I want to go home" can have so many different meanings and that as caregivers we need to be aware of and sensitive to the many shades of meaning such a simple phrase can have. For instance, home could mean safety, security, children, or pets or it could be a person's childhood home or when the person is ready for death (going home to heaven).

Use "yes" to validate how he or she feels, to say I understand and I hear you, and to connect with the person. You can then use "and" to redirect the person and to connect to the person. Try to make polite requests of the person instead of asking questions, which are at times difficult for some people with dementia to answer.

You can find many more examples of using improv and theater in caregiving on Stobbe's website (http://www.in-themoment.com/).

The following are useful tips for caregivers in using improvisation:

Some tips for working with persons with Alzheimer's disease:
Use gestures when trying to get your message across.
Be aware of what your body and face are saying.
Be aware of the tone and inflection of your voice.
Patience is essential.
Join in the person's world, wherever they are. Agree with their reality.
Creativity and flexibility are key.
Avoid situations that bring on anger or frustration.
Break activities and instructions into simple steps.
Avoid quizzing the person and asking questions.
Try to appeal to the person's sense of humor.
Do not argue. Instead of arguing and reasoning, acknowledge and validate.
Acknowledge what is said. Repeat back key points.

Reframe a situation or give the person a new focus.
Orient the person to person, place, and time.
Be flexible. Be ready for anything.
Limit choices to minimize confusion.
Instead of asking questions, give a kind command.
Redirect when possible.
When needed, define your role.

Important characteristics of the caregiver:
Be spontaneous.
Stay focused.
Be nonjudgmental.
Value the moment.
Respect the basic rights of the person.
Use common sense.
Use your sense of humor.
Be flexible.
Maintain optimism.
Set realistic expectations.
Be a good listener.
Communicate skillfully.
Maintain optimism.
Be creative.
Be able to jump into another world.

Some rules of improvisation:
Say "yes" verbally, physically, and mentally.
Listen with your eyes and ears and face.
Stay in the moment.
Always accept a gift.
Don't say "no," say "yes."
Don't ask questions.
Commit to your actions 100%
Combine ideas, even if they are contradictory.
Give focus to those who take it and take focus from those who give it.
Let others define themselves.
Make your actions big.
Don't hesitate; go with the first thought.
Break the rules to move things forward.
Silence can be golden.
Know your audience and show them respect.

Some benefits of improvisation:
Self-confidence
Trust within a group and trust in your own ideas
Teamwork
Listening to others without prejudgment
Breaking from perfectionism
Committing 100%
Letting go of one's own need to control situations or predetermine outcomes
Problem solving
Creativity
Complex thinking; making sense of chaos
Critical thinking; analyzing and relating ideas
Original thinking
A renewing of playfulness
Self-discovery
Expanding limitations

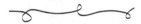

HANDS
MICHELLE OTERO AND THE POETS OF NORTH VALLEY SHARE YOUR CARE

My hands are beautiful.
My hands tell all about life.
My hands touch the birds, the bees, the flowers,
the turnips, the tomatoes and carrots.

My hands are hard and dry because I do all the work
that has to be done, and I love that.
I need a manicure.
The biggest thing my hands did was learn
to send Morse code with a typewriter.
What have my hands done?
Work, play, feelings, holding
hands, raising babies, touching
babies, my dogs, my birds, crocheting, cooking.
They're not tired.
They're ready to go again.

Pass the Smile
With a Sprinkling of Improv Games

Zach, a buzz cut boy of four, smiles.
He smiles his smile unbowed with anything like regret.
Smiles his happiness, nothing dimming him, nothing lost, his only pain
the boy pain of spilt milk and mama mad, smiles his unadorned smile, this
beautiful cherub child, mama milk smile and the room lights up and now
everyone taking Zach's cue, we begin to pass the smile.

The elders, or the Grandpas and Grandmas, as they are referred to in the community of Beneville in Surprise, Arizona, pass Zach's smile to each other and it becomes their smile, their lifetime smile, their seen-it-all smile, their been-there-done-that toothy grin, their jack-o-lantern spooky smile, their kooky laugh-at-it-all smile, and we are laughing, we are all smiling.

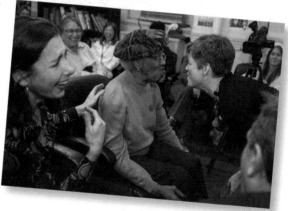

Smiling is contagious, and even if it starts artificially, starts forced after a few smiles, the sunny feeling catches on and we are passing around real smiles, eye-crinkling-at-the-corners smiles, and big sweetheart smiles.

Pass the smile, also known as pass the face or pass the look of shock, is an improv theater game that I learned from Jennie Smith-Peers, executive director of Elder Share the Arts (ESTA) (http://www.estanyc.org/). Smith-Peers is a leader and kindred spirit in the field of dementia arts. Under her direction, ESTA has developed a class using improv at the New York Memory Center (http://nymemorycenter.org/about-us/nymc-in-the-news/).

COUSIN JENNIE'S STEAMING HOT PASS THE SMILE PIE

INGREDIENTS:

2 or more faces (Works best with groups, but you can also be silly and just pass the look back and forth between two people.)

PERFORMANCE TIPS:

If possible, get in a circle or close to a circle. Then one person passes a facial expression to the next person. They repeat it and then pass it off to the next person and so on. When it gets back to the original person, he or she chooses a new facial expression to pass. The object of the game is to build community and trust among the participants.

When working with a group of people living with memory loss, the session leader may need to move around the room as the "face" is passed around, repeating the directions and helping to guide the exercise by demonstrating the gestures.

It is also helpful to reinforce what you are asking them to do: "Bob, now turn to Cathy and smile at her, pass the smile to her." It is natural to compliment the participants on a good smile, and the exercise will often generate a lot of laughter.

UNCLE WILLIAM SHAKESPEARE'S
PASS THE RED BALL AS YOU LIKE IT

INGREDIENTS:

4 or more hands (Works best with groups, but you can also be silly and just pass the look back and forth between two people.)
1 imaginary red ball

PERFORMANCE TIPS:

Instruct the group to gather in a circle. Choose a person to hold the imaginary red ball, then instruct him or her to pass the ball back to the person on his or her right. And then each person in the circle will pass the ball along.

Encourage the group to try to "see" the ball's characteristics as it is passed around. Is the ball heavy? Is the ball light? Does it make a sound? Does it bounce off the ceiling? You get the idea—have a ball with the ball!

Extra Flavor

Add in imaginary balls of other colors and have the participants keep track of what color ball is being passed.

FIVE SENSES PUDDING PARADE

INGREDIENTS:

1 open mind or more, as needed

PERFORMANCE TIPS:

Ask the group to relax and explore their five senses by pretending to:

Touch
- the sun
- a snowball
- a rabbit
- an alligator

Taste
- a bitter, bitter lemon
- their favorite candy
- spinach, broccoli, rattlesnake meat

Hearing
- the wind
- fish singing underwater
- a whistle that only dogs can hear

Sight
- a race car winning the Indy 500
- a giant climbing down a beanstalk
- an ant carrying a leaf
- Little Miss Muffet and her big black spider

Smell
- freshly baked bread
- a stinky skunk
- a French perfume
- freshly chopped onions

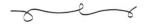

WITHOUT A WORD
JUDY PRESCOTT

Without a word
With a silent plea
A crystal blue yearning
Tongue flipping
You taught me
Without a word
You stayed
One foot in my realm
Steady
Preparing me
You knew
I needed the line
A buoy
You luffed
While waiting
I heard it
This stillness we bandied
Loudly
Beating
Banging
You held
Wings flexed
For the sound
Of my soul
Solid
A sudden shiver
To flight
Without a word
You left me
Full

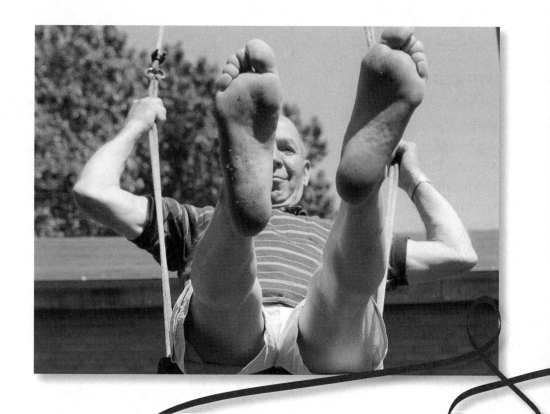

Eight
INTERNATIONAL
PROGRAMMING

The Ducks of Germany
Alle meine Entchen

In September of 2009, the German poets, Lars Ruppel and Dr. Petra Anders, Assistant Professor at Humboldt University of Berlin, invited me to start the Alzheimer's Poetry Project in Germany. As I prepared for my trip, I asked anyone I knew with a connection to Germany about poems and rhymes they had learned as children. While everyone had different suggestions, the one they all shared was the ditty "Alle meine Entchen." This most famous little rhyme that every German knows is not really a poem but a children's song. I have heard it sung on the streets of Berlin by mothers pushing babies in strollers.

Once when I went out on the River Lahn in Marburg, I rowed up to two big construction workers who were welding on a bridge. I said to them, "May I ask you a question, please?" They replied, gruffly, "What? What do you want?" I then began to sing "Alle meine Entchen," and to my delight they joined in, their faces turning into those of two little boys as they sang along.

It is sung to the tune of "I'm a Little Teapot." Shall we give it a try?

Alle meine Entchen
schwimmen auf dem See,
schwimmen auf dem See,
Köpfchen in das Wasser,
Schwänzchen in die Höh.

All my little ducklings,
Swimming on the pond
Swimming on the pond
Heads down in the water
Butt up in the air.

Alzheimer's Poetry Project in Germany

Lars Ruppel is an amazing partner to work with on a poetry project. He was at one time the youngest person making a living as a slam poet, or performance poet, in Germany. He is an amazing organizer, talented performer, and engaging teaching artist. He renamed the Alzheimer's Poetry Project "Weckworte," which translates as "Wake Up Words," an apt description of how the participants react to the poetry.

The APP chapter continues to thrive as Lars incorporates his work teaching poetry slam workshops with bringing students into assisted living centers, or as they are known in Germany, senior houses.

As I had touched on earlier in the book, a poetry slam is a competition during which poets read or recite original work. Previously selected members of the audience then judge the poets' performances on a numeric scale, with 0 being low and 10 being high.

In Germany, many of the poets involved in the APP have ties to the poetry slam movement as well. Germany has the most developed poetry slam scene outside of the United States and their poetry slam events often have attendance in the 100- to 300-person range.

Two slam poets I have trained are Pauline Füg and Henrikje Stanze. Adding to their expertise in doing this work, Füg is also a psychologist and Stanze is a nurse with a master's degree in nursing science. They are work under the name DemenzPoesie. In December 2011, Henrikje came to New York and worked with me when I did a poetry session with Meet Me at MoMA. Much of the work of DemenzPoesie has taken place in museums.

At one of our sessions in Eichstätt, which was organized by Pauline, we created a poem by asking the group what was the most beautiful thing they had seen. We were getting typical responses, such as flowers and sunsets, when a gentleman gave an answer that had clearly caught everyone's attention. My German was not good enough to know what he said, but I felt the energy shift in the room. One of the poets participating in the session, Henrikje Stanze, leaned over and whispered to me, "He just said the most beautiful thing he had ever seen was the day he shot three Russians." Lars moved on and asked the next person what was the most beautiful thing she had ever seen, and in a loud voice she said, "WORLD PEACE!"

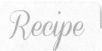

DELICIOUS ALL MY LITTLE DUCKS SOUP

INGREDIENTS:

1 rowboat
2 German construction workers
1 bridge
1 welding torch
1 meandering, slow-flowing river

INSTRUCTIONS:

This recipe works best on a fall day.

1.   Slowly float down the river.

2.   Engage the construction workers with gesticulations and a goofy smile. (Remember, you are a troubadour, carrying the news of poetry from village to village. This is your moment to shine.)

3.   Sing song; repeat as necessary.

Dateline Seoul, South Korea
How a Request for Gangnam Style
Dance Moves to Accompany One of the
Most Revered Korean Poems Almost Started a Riot

One of my goals as a poet is to try as much as possible to bring poetry into everyday life. Upon arriving in South Korea to teach a workshop with project artist Michelle Otero, I had a wonderful opportunity to bridge the language gap with poetry. The driver who picked me up at the airport was chatty and wanted to know what I was doing in South Korea, and my inability to speak Korean was not helping. He understood the words conference and teaching, but when I tried to say "using poetry," I lost him. Then I remembered I had poem translations with me and that they were in English and Korean. As traffic allowed, I handed him a poem and as he read

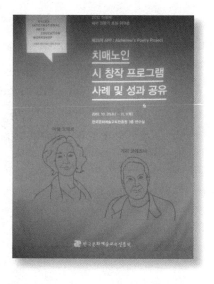

it, the language gap was finally bridged. He knew the poem and understood I was using poetry to work with elders. He loved reading the poem for me, and I loved that as we crept through the streets of Seoul I was hearing the poem in its native language.

As I checked into the hotel, the lesson repeated. "What brings you to Seoul?" This time I immediately shared the poem with the young women at the desk, who began laughing—they understood I wanted them to perform the poem as a trio and in unison. The hotel lobby was alive as they performed the poem.

For the workshop, I had decided to use the well-known Korean poem "Azaleas," by Kim Sowol. During the workshop, I had asked if they would mind putting some Gangnam style dance moves to "Azaleas." (The pop song

"Gangnam Style" and the dance named after it, which is made up of a series of horse trots, were popularized internationally in 2012 by the Korean musician Psy.) I immediately knew by the looks of horror and audible gasps that I had made a huge mistake. I tried to take it back, but nothing would stop the avalanche of comments erupting from the students. The translator was struggling to keep up with the wave of suggestions and what I could do with my brilliant idea.

Slowly, I was able to calm them and we agreed that while Gangnam style was out of the question, the group would try improvising to the poem in a manner more in keeping with the tone of the poem, which describes a time in Korean history when Japan occupied Korea, and the azaleas serve as a symbol of the people's sadness. (You can see the dance and hear the poem being performed in Korean by logging on to http://www.youtube.com/watch?v = Pw_Q9FdVN0Q)

Below is a wonderful translation of "Azaleas" by Brother Anthony, who was extremely generous in providing me with Korean-to-English translation of some of the most well-known and well-loved Korean poems.

진달래꽃 (김소월)	AZALEAS BY KIM SO-WŎL
나 보기가 역겨워 가실 때에는 말없이 고이 보내 드리오리다. 영변(寧邊)에 약산(藥山) 진달래꽃, 아름 따다 가실 길에 뿌리오리다. 가시는 걸음 걸음 놓인 그 꽃을 사뿐히 즈려★ 밟고 가시옵소서. 나 보기가 역겨워 가실 때에는 죽어도 아니 눈물 흘리오리다.	When seeing me sickens you and you walk out I'll send you off without a word, no fuss. Yongbyon's mount Yaksan's azaleas by the armful I'll scatter in your path. With parting steps on those strewn flowers treading lightly, go on, leave. When seeing me sickens you and you walk out why, I'd rather die than weep one tear.

Cake Boy Parties Down at the U.S. Embassy in Warsaw

How to Write a Superhero Poem

A school bus in Warsaw is full of kids who are all yelling "Cake Boy, Cake Boy," calling out Bohdan Piasecki's poetry superhero name, like he is a famous rock star and they are his loving fans. At this moment, Bohdan is a bit of a poetry rock star, and he signs his autograph for all of them.

I imagine the kids at home that night sharing around the dinner table: "You won't believe it, but today we met a real poet and I got his autograph and he taught us how to write superhero poems, and then we went to an Alzheimer's home and shared poetry with the people who live there and we all laughed and smiled and it was so fun, and, Mom, can I be a poet when I grow up?"

We are in Poland and the Alzheimer's Poetry Project is translating with ease into the language and culture. How did we get to Poland? Well, sometimes it is who you know or, even better, who knows you. When my sister-in-law, Carmen Victor, moved with her sweet family to Poland, little did I know it would lead to a pilot project for APP funded by the U.S. Embassy in Warsaw. Carmen's son, Rex, was in the same class as the son of the U.S. Ambassador and they often played together. It was easy for Carmen to chat about her brother-in-law's amazing work through APP with representatives at the U.S. Embassy in Berlin. One thing led to another, and soon I was submitting a proposal to the program director. Of course, we had to win the contract on our own merit, but what Carmen did was ensure that the right person saw the proposal.

By the Numbers

APP's Polish pilot project took place over a period of 7 days in April 2012 with 11 events, including training sessions, workshops, classroom poetry lessons, public readings, and a school assembly in Warsaw and Krakow. A total of 730 people participated, including:

- 119 people living with Alzheimer's disease or a related dementia

- 22 healthcare workers

- 495 students (assembly sessions and two classroom workshops)

- 12 teachers

- 7 poets

In addition, 75 people from the general public attended an event that was held at the rock club Kosmos Kosmos in Warsaw to hear stories and poems about the project. The healthcare workers, students, teachers, and poets received training in how to engage people living with memory loss in the performance and creation of poetry.

Intergenerational Programming

One of the highlights of working in Poland was the chance to bring students from the American School in Warsaw to a local assisted living center to perform and create poems with the residents. A group of local poets and I, including the lead artist of the project and an amazing translator, Bohdan Piasecki, went to the school to work with the students from Ms. Gruzen's 2nd grade class. To give you a sense of Piasecki's translation skills, if you watched the Academy Awards in Poland, it was Piasecki's voice you heard. He was part of the simultaneous translation crew for the broadcast.

The school administration had arranged for us to perform poetry as part of a school-wide assembly for 500 students. In preparation for the assembly, the students wrote original poems in the voices of superheroes and modeled on Bohdan's poem, "Cake Boy." The students created their characters as well as gave them super powers and a motto. Students from Ms. Gruzen's class performed the poems for the assembly. The following are a few of the students' poems.

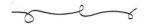

CHOCOLATE GIRL
ZOSHA

Chocolate, Chocolate, Chocolate, Chocolate Girl!
Chocolate here, Chocolate there, Chocolate everywhere!
Rain of Chocolate, bath of Chocolate!
Motto: Don't forget to eat some Chocolate for breakfast!

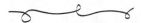

EAT YOUR VEGGIES, MAN
REX

Shoot peas out of hands.
Grow atomic bell peppers.
Make veggies appear out of nowhere.
Fly on a jet-powered pickle.
Very good at veggie food fights.
Has superhero veggie strength.
Motto: Don't forget to eat your veggies, man.

The students created poems in English and Polish and they also learned how to perform poems and public-speaking skills. They were given instruction on Alzheimer's disease and related dementias and what to expect during their field trip to the assisted living center. After the visit, they wrote about their experiences in working with people living with memory loss.

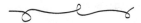

AT THE ALZHEIMER CENTER
ALEXIA

Looking
At the older people
My eyes
Are filled with
Tears
That disease is
Very
Bad
I think
While sitting

On the hard
Cement floor
I am so
Nervous
And amazed
With the
Poetry
They say
While Bohdan says
The poetry
And they follow
Along

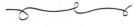

TRIP TO THE ALZHEIMER CENTER
MARC

Driving on the bus
Very long.
In the lobby
Two old men
On the black sofa
Calm and peaceful!

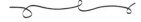

THE ALZHEIMER CENTER
OLIVER

I looked
Terrified!
When I got there
I saw small people, big people
Some had wrinkles
Some were in wheelchairs
I really was amazed
When we read poetry
I thought they couldn't
even remember
Yesterday!
They laughed!
I thought they never would.
That was the miracle!

Dichos
Spanish-Language Programming

"My father would never let me kiss boys, but my father wasn't always there," a woman says to me as we create a poem about first kisses. Everyone has a first kiss story. Another woman says, "We never even kissed. My boyfriend and I only held hands." Everyone in the room sighs at learning this. A man says, "I would wait by the river and my girlfriend would walk down to get water for her family and we would kiss."

Try to picture in your mind the next person to answer: a tiny woman, not even 5-feet tall, in her 90s, thin and frail and with a regal bearing, perched in her chair as if it were a throne. She points to her cheek and says, "He kissed me here." She points to her lips and says, "He kissed me here." She then draws herself up, back straight, and as she slowly draws an imaginary line across her neck says, "I told him, you don't kiss me below here." She beams like a queen as her subjects burst with laughter.

The dynamic Nelva Olin, program coordinator of the Latino Geriatric Center in Milwaukee, Wisconsin, led the hour-long session I just described. The Alzheimer's Poetry Project was expanding our Spanish-language programming, which had begun in Santa Fe, New Mexico, to better serve people living with dementia whose first language is Spanish.

We had had success in our Spanish-language programming in the use of *dichos*, or folk sayings that are passed mouth to ear, from one generation to the next. They serve as advice, or warnings, and are often funny. *Dichos* are similar to haiku in length and in passing on wisdom, and we have found a high level of response to them from people living with dementia.

Olin began by using the APP technique of call and response by saying a line of the *dicho* and then asking the group to repeat after her:

Pan es pan, queso es queso
no hay amor sino hay un beso.

Bread is bread, cheese is cheese
Without a kiss there is no love.

The program director, Al Castor, remembered as a child this particular *dicho* being used as a rhyme that kids would jump rope to. Using the *dicho* and laughing at the words warmed up the group. Olin continued by asking each person to talk about his or her first kiss. This led to an enthusiastic response from each of the 12 participants. The stories and the laughter were contagious. Some talked about how food was scarce and that while cheese and bread were hard to come by, their mothers' kisses kept them full. In general, each person would describe his or her first kiss and then he or she would use the structure of the *dicho* to add an image to the poem. You can see some of their responses used as lines in the following poem.

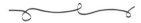

KISSES

No affection or kisses.
When I was a child,
I would ask my parents for bread and cheese.
They could not give it to me.
But they could give me love.

My first boyfriend, we only held hands.

Love is greater than bread and cheese.
When I went to the store,
there was no bread or cheese.
But I found a girl to kiss.

I would wait down by the river,
my girlfriend would come to get water for her family,
then we would kiss.

Girls don't kiss me.
They reject me.
No one ever loved me.
Only my mother loved me a bit.
My mother said, "I'll give you bread and cheese,
and if you don't eat these
I won't kiss you."

This means that if you have a boyfriend or a girlfriend
and you don't kiss them
you won't get bread either.

I told him,
you can kiss me here.
(she points to her cheek)
You can kiss me here.
(she points to her lips)
But you don't kiss me below here.
(She draws a line across her chin)

When you are a teenager
At 14, 15, or 16, you dream a lot
But at 18 you already know
to say yes or no,
then you can eat your dessert.

Nútreme Hoy (Nurture Me Today)

In 2010, APP's Spanish-language anthology was published *Nútreme Hoy* (*Nurture Me Today*). It includes 50 poems and *dichos*, as well as essays on how to use poetry to connect to people living with dementia and how to create a poetry program. (For more information on APP's Spanish-language programming, visit http://www.alzpoetry.com/Nutreme%20Hoy/)

While doing research for *Nútreme Hoy* at the Fray Angélico Chávez History Library in Santa Fe, I came across a treasure trove of Spanish-language newspapers that had once flourished in New Mexico. The librarians pointed out to me the book *Spanish-Language Newspapers in New Mexico, 1834–1958*, by Gabriel Meléndez. One of the things that excited me was that the editors often published poems and gave them prominence on the first page of the paper. I loved looking at the old papers on microfiche and feeling like a time traveler. My Spanish is limited, but the look of a poem on a page is universal, and so when I thought I had come across one, I would print it out and show it to the librarians, who would confirm for me that it was, indeed, a poem.

One poem I was most excited about was "Analysis of the Parts that Comprise a Kiss," which was written by the most famous poet of all time, Anonymous. I knew immediately that it was a poem, and with *beso* in the title meant that it was probably a poem about kissing. Below is the poem as it appears in *Nútreme Hoy* and in its original Spanish translation by our talented translator, Anacelie Verde Claro. Tradition has it that publishing it anonymously probably meant it was written by the editor of the paper, which would have been an open secret for the readers. See if this little bit of New Mexico history also feels to you like a recipe for a kiss:

Analysis of the Parts that Comprise a Kiss
ANONYMOUS

Drop of nectar, good and pure,
Drip of ambrosia on it—
Gram or two of rhyming sonnet,
Half note from an overture.

Bead of honey dripping slow—
Powdered fly, well, just a speck,
With something else magnetic,
Flavor of an open rose.

Atom of sheer modesty—
Four ounces more of tenderness,
Other sorts of craziness,
A scruple of love, naturally.

Análisis de las partes de que se compone un beso
ANÓNIMO

De nectar puro—una gota,
Un adarme de ambrosía—
Un gramo de la poesía,
De música media nota.

Una gotita de miel—
De cantárida—un polvito,
De magnetismo—un tantito,
Sabor de rosa y clavel.

Un átomo de pudor—
Cuatro dracmas de ternura,
Otras tantas de locura—
Y un escrúpulo de amor.

International Programming

Our goal through the Alzheimer's Poetry Project is to have the methods and techniques we have developed and successfully used be translated into every language and culture. Having already had our approach beautifully translated into German, Hmong, Hebrew, Korean, Mandarin, Polish, and Spanish and having conducted sessions internationally in Australia, Germany, Poland, and South Korea have made us want to pursue this lofty goal. In each case we have identified well-loved and well-known poems from diverse cultures to use with people living with memory loss.

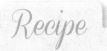

WORLD POETRY STEW

INGREDIENTS:

1 poet knowledgeable in the poetry of his or her native language and culture (If possible, the person should also be a strong organizer and have a large network of poets and friends.)

1 heaping source of funding

1 prime cut translator (This person can be the above-mentioned poet or they can work together.)

1 cauldron

1 giant ladle

1 dream

1 eye of newt

INSTRUCTIONS:

Bring cauldron to boil. Slowly stir the ingredients together, moving the ladle in a clockwise direction while chanting: "Double, double boil, toil, and trouble, fire burn and cauldron bubble. Cross fingers, knock on wood, wink eye of newt, let the steam rise up and carry this message, wandering lonely as a cloud until your heart with pleasure fills and you dance with the dollar bills from on high." You must dream it first.

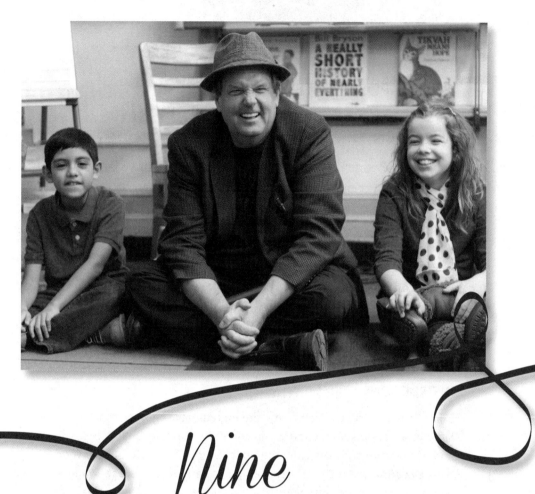

Nine
INTERGENERATIONAL
PROGRAMMING

Poetry for Life

When I speak to people about using poetry with older adults, one of the comments I hear again and again is that while the generation that preceded the baby boomers learned poetry in school, with most having memorized some poems by heart as part of their education, the baby boomer generation for the most part did not. People always ask what will happen as the pre–baby boomer generation passes away and fewer and fewer people recognize classic poems.

My strongest answer to that question is that the poems we use from the Elizabethan era, including those from the bard, the rhyme champion, and in a way the inventor of the inner life of the human mind, our dear Shakespeare, are over 400 years old. And the poems of the law-firm-sounding team of Wordsworth, Keats, Coleridge, and Shelly are from the Romantic era of over 200 years ago. So, will they soon be forgotten? Will they be disappearing from our consciousness in the near future? Not likely.

Consider, for example, the generation of today and the influence of hip-hop on cultures worldwide. You can enter a classroom and at least some of the students are deeply into writing lines that rhyme and have rhythm. It is a golden time to write rhythm and rhyme.

The Alzheimer's Poetry Project started with a moment of inspiration when a man, seemingly unaware of life going on around him, heard a poem being recited, finished a line of the poem, and, like magic, began participating with the rest of the group. While this happens on a regular basis as part of our sessions, and when it does happen it is truly inspirational, the fact is that it is less than 5 percent of the APP experience.

Most people do not know poems by heart, and so that moment of recollection is not going to happen for them. Most people are responding to the performance the teaching artist is sharing with them. They are responding to that person's enthusiasm, to the joy he or she is bringing to the lesson. They are sharing an experience with their peers. They are bonding with them and the teaching artist in the sheer love of language and that will never change, no matter which current and future generations we are serving.

Poetry for Life Project

This brings us to the Poetry for Life (PFL) project. I am not going to sit on my hands and worry about people not learning poems by heart. I launched the PFL project in partnership with the Poetry Foundation and with funding from the Alzheimer's Foundation of America and the Pabst Charitable Foundation of the Arts. PFL is a pilot project that joins the skills and passion of the young poets of the Poetry Out Loud: National Recitation Contest with older adults in adult day centers or who reside in assisted living. In addition, PFL will offer training for teaching artists and healthcare workers to deepen their knowledge of using poetry to improve the quality of life of people living with Alzheimer's disease and related dementia by facilitating creative expression through poetry. PFL seeks to bring the power of recited poetry to this under-served segment of our community.

In 2013, 375,000 students participated in the Poetry Out Loud national recitation contest, which is structured like a spelling bee, with a participant winning at the classroom level and then school-, city-, and state-level champion. In April of each year, all 52 states and territories send a winner to Washington, D.C., and one student advances to that year's champion and wins a $20,000 scholarship. Even if only 5 to 10 percent of students participate in Poetry for Life, that means 20,000 to 40,000 young poets volunteering to perform and create poems with older adults in assisted living, adult day, and senior centers. It will change the scope of arts engagement for older adults across the nation.

PFL held its first session at Sunnyside High School in Tucson, Arizona, with their Poetry Club under the direction of teacher extraordinaire Kurt Fischer. Long-time friends and poets Matthew John Conley and Logan Phillips, who are teaching artists for the University of Arizona Poetry Center for Poetry Out Loud, also attended the meeting. The students were excited about the training they received, and I think it bodes well for the success of the project that this group was there from day one.

We held the second session in partnership with Banu Valladares, Arts in Education Director, North Carolina Arts. One of the students, Jacquim Strickland from Andrews High School in High Point, said about his experience,

> We went to the nursing home to perform Poetry Out Loud. It was mind blowing to see how we could relate, even though we were in different circumstances and different ages, how we could all come together and connect. It was good communication. You get someone to respond to you that has a disability. It shows you that they are listening and they want something to do.

PFL Program Design

The PFL program will have two major components:

1. Teaching artists and healthcare workers will receive training in reciting poetry using materials developed by Poetry Out Loud and posted to their website (http://www.poetryoutloud.org). They will also learn APP techniques and methods. We completed the healthcare worker component of the pilot project, which was held in Appleton, Wisconsin, and it was a smash success! The Poetry Out Loud materials focus on building public-speaking and performance skills, including projection, articulation, pacing of the recitation, dynamics, and bringing out the emotional content of the poem.

2. Schools participating in the Poetry Out Loud national recitation contest are matched with an assisted living facility or adult day or senior center. Initial meetings take place between the project director, teachers, and facility staff to plan the workshops.

APP On-line Training Session

You, too, can participate and receive the same preparation described above through APP's on-line training and certification workshop. (For more information, log on to http://www.alzpoetry.com/On-Line%20Training/) This book is the textbook that is used to lead the training, so you are already participating! This fun, high-energy on-line training is an opportunity to deepen your skills as a caregiver, healthcare professional, or teaching artist, and is packed full of simple techniques to create and perform poems with people living dementia and to help develop high-quality arts programs for them.

As part of the on-line training, you will learn:

*   How to structure an arts program for people living with memory loss

*   How to perform and create poetry with people living with Alzheimer's disease and a related dementia in both the home and facility settings

*   How to use art to engage people in group discussions that are used to create poetry, stories, or songs

Recipe

CHANGE THE WORLD POETRY PIE

INGREDIENTS:

1 stubborn poet
1 lifetime of work
1 billion minds

INSTRUCTIONS:

Simmer on low for a long time, stir gently, and change the world one mind at a time.

Kids Playing with Words

In 1968 at Olive Elementary School in Novato, California, my sixth-grade teacher, Mr. White, read to us from *The Hobbit* every day after lunch. I want to set the time period and place because Novato is 30 miles north of San Francisco, it is the late 1960s, and the Grateful Dead are living commune style at Rancho Olompali just a few miles north of the school. This is the time and place I mark as the development of my creative imagination. I have strong memories of walking home from school replaying the day's story after listening to Mr. White enthrall us with the tales of hobbits, dragons, elves, and magic rings of invisibility and immense power:

> One Ring to rule them all, One Ring to find them,
> One Ring to bring them all and in the darkness bind them

Heady stuff for a boy of 10! It felt rural and wild on those walks home along a worn path through the grass and gullies carved out by the rain, where later would be sidewalks and more formal streets. At the house next to the school you could watch a rancher shear his sheep and climb up the orchard trees and pick fresh plums or peaches. The rancher made his own olive oil next door to Olive Elementary School. The streets around the school lived up to the names of Cherry, Plum, and Peach Streets.

It was rural, it was woolly, and it was wild. Soon I would start to go to concerts and catch the tail end of the 1960s, but for then it was enough to be a boy soaking up all of the rural wildness. Novato was a beautiful place to grow up.

As I walked, I would reimagine and see in my mind's eye the battles in *The Hobbit*. Mr. White reading to us made me fall in love with words. And I was so thrilled that the words could fuel stories of my own and that my imagination could make them come alive.

This love of words and stories is what I bring to my work with kids, or, as I love to call them, "the young knowledge seekers." One of the biggest honors I have had in working with youth was having been asked to give the graduation speech for ACE Preschool in Brooklyn, New York. It is so sweet and funny to think of the little 4 and 5 year-olds graduating from preschool to kindergarten. The following are the poem and speech I wrote for the event:

> As you go forth into the world and think "what does the future hold for me?," remember you have a very important job to do and that job as children is to play!

Children teach us how to play.
They remind us to say, make time to play.
Okay, we say, Okay, Okay, time to play!
What shall we do today?
Shall we play?
Shall we swim in a bay?
Shall we feed a horse some hay?
What if the horse says neigh?
Can you lead a horse to a eat a buffet?
Can you teach the horse to crochet?
Of course, of course, you say!
Olé! Olé! Olé! Olé!
Make way, make way, its time to play.
Would a horse sniff a flower bouquet?
Would that horse eat a chocolate soufflé?
And wash it down with a café au lait?
You taught us all how to play
Now we say, we say, we say
Happy, Happy, Happy Graduation Day!
Happy Graduation Day to you!

> I have been working with these young knowledge seekers since 2012, teaching them to perform poetry. After they learn a poem, we then go downstairs to meet our neighbors at the New York Memory Center. We share the poems with the older adults, and we often create poems with them as well. Together we share laughter as friends. Now when I arrive at New York Memory Center to do a session, the people who are navigating memory loss will ask me, "Where are the kids? Go get the kids!" These are people living with Alzheimer's disease who so strongly remember the students' visits that they say to me, "Don't come without the kids!"

Children remind us of the good in the world. They remind us to slow down, to live, and to enjoy life. As the job of a child is to play, they also remind us to play and to enjoy a laugh and share a smile. When playing, kids imagine, and through their imaginations they teach us how to find laughter and joy in the world. At the end of the day, as they drift off to sleep, they remind us to dream, and through their dreams and in their faces, smiles, and laughter we see the future. Let us praise the play and dreams and imagination of children and thank them for what they teach us. Together let us wish them a Happy Graduation!

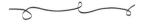

(From "Recipe to Make Us Younger," created with the elders at Barelas–Share Your Care in Albuquerque, NM)

Start with sugar.
Put it in the pot.

Echa soledad.

More sugar.

Nobody can make us younger.
We get older every year.

More sugar.

Cook it in the oven and cut it.

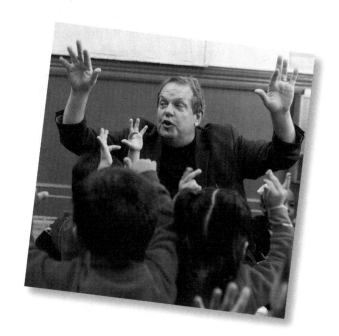

TIO GARY'S OLD-TIMEY WORD GAME

INGREDIENTS:

2 hands
1 happy face
1 big mouth

INSTRUCTIONS:

This is a poem, or as we often say when working with preschool kids, a game with words. It is a simple lesson on saying "hello." Begin by saying: "We are going to play a game. I am going to say a word and I want you to say what I say. I say 'it'! You say 'it'! Ready? Please let me see your eyes when you are ready. Look at me so I know you are listening and ready. Good! Good! I say 'it,' then you say 'it.' Here we go." At a certain point in every class with preschool kids I say "cheese burger." For some reason this makes everyone laugh. At various times throughout the performance of the "Hello" poem, I will blast in with a hearty shout of "cheese burger!" Or I will growl or howl "cheese burger" like a dog.

continued

HELLO

It's time to say hello!
hello, hello, hello, hello, hello, hello.

These are my hands
that wave in the air!

These are my hands
that point to the sky!

These are my hands
I wave them high!

hello, hello, hello, hello, hello, hello.

hello, hello, hello, hello, hello, hello.

These are my hands
that wave in the air!

These are my hands
that point to the sky!

These are my hands
I wave them high!

hello, hello, hello, hello, hello, hello.

hello, hello, hello, hello, hello, hello.

Good morning, everybody!
It's a good, good day!

hello, hello, hello, hello, hello, hello.

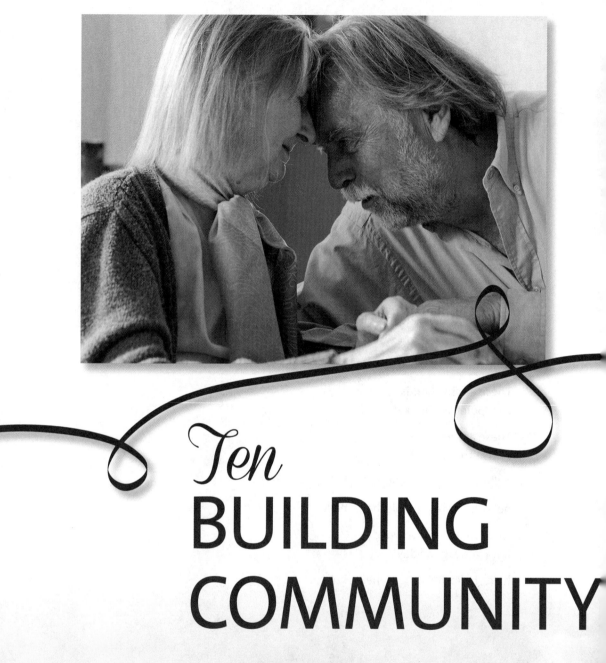

Ten
BUILDING
COMMUNITY

Through the Looking Glass— A Lesson in Empathy

I am sitting in a wheelchair, my adult diaper full of vanilla pudding.

This is the climax—the moment I have been waiting for. And after a few minutes, I can barely feel the wet, cold pudding. You can get used to anything.

In a strange take on the writer's retreat, I chose to live for a week in a skilled nursing home as part of an innovative program called Through the Looking Glass. Developed in 2009 by Leslie Pedtke, the program is designed to teach empathy to staff who care for people living with dementia at Aviston Countryside Manor in Illinois. I had met Leslie at a Pioneer Network Conference, learned about the program, and asked if I could take part.

Through the Looking Glass helps the staff learn what it is like to *live* in the place where they work, a place I learned firsthand is so full of love and caring and fully reflects Leslie's desire and drive to run a perfect nursing home.

Leslie Pedtke on Through the Looking Glass

(Gary) Please tell us what inspired you.

(Leslie) "In 2009, I came up with the idea of having the staff move in and live as residents. I was sitting one morning with a woman who was dying. The door was shut and it was quiet in her room, just she and I. She was not responding to me; I am not sure she was aware I was even there.

"Hearing life continue on just outside her door, I wondered what Lila thought of us. What her last few months with us were like. If she felt like we treated her well, if she enjoyed her life here. What her life was like as a little girl, and growing up. When she met her first boyfriend. Was she thinking of all of those things while she was dying? I wondered if the staff could ever grasp what it was like to be Lila."

(Gary) *I love the idea of understanding what it was like to be Lila. What did you do next?*

(Leslie) After I left her room, I asked some of the staff members what they thought of the idea of having the staff move in and live as residents at Aviston. At the time, the television show 'Survivor' was really popular, and I thought it could be like the show—every day we could involve challenges that our *residents* face every day, challenges that we think are no big deal but are a really big deal to them. Like being incontinent and having to eat puréed food, needing someone to wait on you when it comes to basic needs like having to go to the bathroom, not being able to do that by yourself."

(Gary) *How has the program been received?*

(Leslie) "Through the Looking Glass has been an overwhelming success, and made us who we are. Staff members who haven't participated still learn from the people who have participated.

"One of the participants, Amy, received a diagnosis of blindness, and we have a gentleman here who is blind. We learn from Amy as an example and ask her, 'How did it feel? How do you think he is feeling?' We ask if people are restless in their wheelchairs, and how did it feel to be in that wheelchair? 'It sucked. My legs were tired after only being in the chair for an hour.'

"It gives people something to think about when they listen to what their co-workers went through, because sometimes we look at the resident and think, 'I don't know what to do about that.' Or if it is someone who can't communicate with us, asking co-workers what they think from personal experience adds credibility."

A Tisket, a Tasket, a Challenged-Filled Basket

"How would you like to live in a Looking-glass House, Kitty? I wonder if they'd give you milk in there? Perhaps looking-glass milk isn't any good to drink—"

—Alice, *Through the Looking Glass*

For each day of the program, Leslie brings a basket filled with strips of paper. Written on each strip is a challenge, such as "Your incontinence has caused you to soak your pants with urine," "Speech therapy recommends puréed food for one meal," or "Your caregiver will feed you lunch today." It is like getting a fortune cookie, only the fortune is always bad.

As part of my experience of Through the Looking Glass, Leslie and her staff have decided to not make my diagnosis as bad as others they give out, and to take it easy on me with the challenges. One of their staff, for example, received a diagnosis of blindness and had to wear goggles that distorted her sight. My challenge was pretty easy compared to that one. I am given a diagnosis of a stroke. I spend the week in a wheelchair. My left arm is strapped down to the arm of the chair, and weights are placed on my left leg to help mimic the loss of movement.

Pudding Pants

And once she had really frightened her old nurse by shouting suddenly in her ear, "Nurse! Do let's pretend that I'm a hungry hyena and you're a bone . . . "

—Alice, *Through the Looking Glass*

Leslie handed me the adult diaper and the cans of pudding (yes, plural, cans!). She leaves me and I take my time putting on my nappy. To get the full effect, I head into the main room and spend time talking with people. It feels strange, but, of course, no one notices.

Soaked with the sticky-sweet dessert, I wheel back to the bathroom to clean up. I feel relief, and a small sense of letdown that I have so easily passed the pudding pants challenge.

The bathrooms are shared, and have doors that open to both rooms to allow you to enter from either side. Once inside you easily hear anything being said in the rooms next door. As I take off my pudding-soaked diaper, a man in the next room yells, "Quit playing with my balls! If you want to play with someone's balls, get a dog. My balls, my balls, my balls, quit playing with my balls. Listen sister, you're not playing with my balls. I had it out with your sisters last week, and I'll have it out with you this week. My balls, my balls, my balls, quit playing with my balls."

The Certified Nursing Assistant (CNA) answers back, "We are not playing with your balls!"

Any sense I have of "this is easy" and "having pudding in my pants is a breeze" is smacked by the ferocity of his cry—"My balls! Ass on fire, my balls!" The man's anger, confusion, and disorientation fill me as full as the vanilla pudding adult diaper I am staring down at.

The rich language slaps my ears, slaps my brain, giving me a good whack upside the head. It brings me back to that first moment long ago, delivering flowers and hearing people cry out for help. It is why I began creating poetry with people living with dementia, and it scares the shit out of me—the real shit, not the fake pudding kind.

I know they are not playing with his balls. Still, his pain is real in a way that my pretending at having incontinence is not. He cannot distinguish between real and not real; he has slipped through the looking glass.

The CNA remains calm and talks to him in a soothing voice. She respects and acknowledges what he is saying, but redirects him in order to finish her task. This is a clear and strong example of working under pressure, keeping your cool, and remaining professional, even while being unfairly yelled at.

While Leslie's dream of running a *perfect* nursing home may never be attained, she and everyone at Aviston should never stop trying for that goal. We should all follow their example.

As the man relaxed and responded to her voice and manner, the CNA took his worst moment of fear, confusion, and anger and made it right. *That* is perfect.

The next day I asked Amy, the Assistant Director of Nursing, about the situation. Here is what she said:

> We are working with a population that has dementia. They forget who we are every day. Even though we see them every day and we remember them, they forget who we are every few hours, if not every few minutes. We need to remind ourselves to explain a procedure. Even though we just did five minutes ago, they have probably forgotten, and that is terrifying to them.
>
> Why is this stranger trying to get into my private area? It could feel scary to them and traumatic. So the staff needs to be very explanatory, very thorough and have a lot of patience, because even though you explained it five minutes ago, you need to explain it again and again and again. They just don't remember.

As the days flowed and everything I was experiencing began to blend, I looked forward to the challenges.

Being Fed

I draw, "Your caregiver will feed you lunch today," so I have to pretend that I cannot feed myself. I sit at the "feeders' table." The act of being fed is not so bad. What makes this almost unbearable is how the other feeders look at you with a mixture of solidarity and confusion. At times during my week of Through the Looking Glass, feelings of being a fraud rise. These are some of the hardest moments.

I do not want to make fun of the residents, and I do not want my playing this game to be disrespectful. And my natural way of dealing with stressful situations is to use humor to make a joke.

At first I try this with Brenda, but laughing at the feeder table feels forced, and so I start just to nod when Brenda asks me if I am ready for another bite. Like the other feeders, I nod, take the spoon into my mouth, and eat my food. Throughout the week my constant mantra—you can get used to anything.

The Truth About Playing Bingo

"How puzzling all these changes are! I'm never sure what I'm going to be, from one minute to another."
—Alice, *Through the Looking Glass*

We play bingo sometimes two times a day. Is my brain slowing down? Is it possible I can *feel* my brain slow down? After an hour of bingo, it sure feels like it is. This is the moment I feel most institutionalized, and many people have pointed out that bingo is not the most creative of activities.

Drawing the challenges gives a structure to my time here and I have used that structure in this essay. The structure here includes meal times and physical therapy, but there is a drifting quality to time here and a *déjà vu* or Ground Hog Day feeling to the repetition of days in a skilled nursing home. There is also a feeling of slipping through the looking glass and entering into another world. This is never stronger than when I play bingo, with its repetitive calling of numbers and playing multiple games.

On the flip side, I feel so good when I win. A real elation and feeling of joy comes over me, even while I know, intellectually, that it is not a great accomplishment to win bingo. How must it feel to live here? When a person living here wins, it is a real win. I am getting used to bingo and looking forward to bingo, and in a major shift in my thinking of the virtues of this game, bingo is a big part of my day.

All ears listen for the next call, shushing and hushing, the silence in the room amplifying their focused attention, this room full of elders—long-ago teachers, bakers, farmer's wives, now serious players of bingo who brook no distractions, no idle gossip, no talking unless you are the caller saying, "B4."

A huge plus in playing bingo is that the elders watch out for each other. The people who have a hard time hearing the numbers being called, or focusing long enough to follow whether their numbers have been called, are helped by the others. Some are gently reminded that they have a number, gently helped to place the marker on the right square, gently told that they, in fact, have bingo, and helped to cry out, bingo! In helping those who need help, you become a bingo expert, and to be an expert is a good thing.

"Tell them you have bingo."

"I have bingo?"

"Yes, say bingo."

"Bingo!"

Getting to Know All About You

The Mad Hatter: "Have I gone mad?"

Alice: "I'm afraid so. You're entirely bonkers. But I'll tell you a secret. All the best people are."

—Through the Looking Glass

At first drawing, "You coughed a little on your nectar-thick drinks at breakfast and need to increase to honey thick," it seemed to be a pretty easy challenge. I drank down my thickened coffee at breakfast. It was a little sweet and strange, but not bad at all. At lunch I enjoyed my thickened juice. It was only after a couple of days that I began to notice I was constipated. In a skilled nursing home, bowel movements are a regular topic of discussion, so I fit right in.

As I lie in bed, I begin a little mantra in my head, my inner voice chanting: I am constipated. I am never constipated. Am I going crazy? I am constipated. I am never constipated. Can just being here drive you crazy? I am constipated. I am never constipated. I am constipated. I am never constipated. Can just being here drive you crazy?

I say to my roommate, "Andy, I am constipated. I'm never constipated. I think it's all the thickened liquids I've been drinking."

"You should try chocolate milk."

He tells me his theory of chocolate milk: "You should drink chocolate milk with every meal. Chocolate milk is delicious and it keeps you regular. It's important to keep regular. Chocolate milk is nutritious and delicious. I love my chocolate milk."

I begin to grab other people's waters at mealtime and drink them down before the staff can stop me. I chug down water and leave my thickened drinks untouched.

As embarrassed as I am about being constipated, I finally screw up my courage and tell Leslie. Without batting an eyelash, she takes me off thickened liquids. Perfect.

On my last day, I tell Andy what it has meant to be his roommate, how I have enjoyed his sense of humor. We are both lying in our beds and on the wall is a mirror, a looking glass, and we can see each other, without turning to the side. As I pour my heart out, Andy cracks a wicked grin and sings, "Getting to know you, getting to know all about you . . . "

Irma and Billy and My Wet Pants

When I draw, "Your incontinence has caused you to soak your pants with urine," the staff enlists Irma to pour water on my lap to mimic loss of bladder control. Although I know I will be faced with this challenge, I do not know *when* it will happen. I am out in the common area reading the newspaper when Irma sneaks up on me.

I see Irma out of the corner of my eye: she has a pitcher full of water and pours some of it on me. It is cold, but not bad. Then she gets a glint in her eye and, laughing, she dumps the full pitcher directly onto my crotch. Now it is cold, and I am soaked.

After the initial shock wears off, I realize I have to change my clothes and take my soiled pants to the laundry. Luckily, one of the aides is going by and I explain what has happened. She wheels me to my room to change, and then I wheel myself down to the laundry and the aide there helps me put my clothes in the dryer.

At each step, as I have to explain again what has happened, I feel the shame of having soiled myself. Even though we are playing Through the Looking Glass and none of this is real, it feels real. The shame and emotion are real.

For the rest of the day, every time Irma sees me she says, "Why did they make me do that? Why did they make me pour water on you?"

Billy is Irma's best friend here. It feels a lot like high school, where certain people gravitate to each other and hang out. Billy wears blue jean overalls, which reminds me of the way many of my farmer relatives from Oklahoma dress.

I start hanging out with Billy and Irma. One of my Through the Looking Glass social highlights is staying up late with them and a few others and watching their beloved Saint Louis Cardinals baseball team on television. There is a Through the Looking Glass moment when the announcer says, "I want to thank all of our fans watching in nursing homes." We look at each other, laugh, high-five, and say, "Hey, the television is talking to us!"

Spy in the House of Old

Through my participation in Through the Looking Glass, I learned compassion, to slow down, what it *feels* like to slow down, and what being bored really feels like. And this brings me to the hardest moment of my stay at Aviston: saying good-bye to Mimi.

I met Mimi at breakfast my second or third day at Aviston. She was funny and quiet and recognized that, like her, I had my arm strapped down. Like her I was in a wheelchair, and like her I was in my mid-fifties. After breakfast, we both sat in the main room, uninterested in attending the church service going on in the activity room.

I wheel over near her and ask if I can ask her a question. She says, "Sure." I take out my notebook and pen and get ready to write. I can tell she is curious about me carrying a notebook, so I tell her, "I am writing about staying here to help me get a sense of what it is like to live here. May I ask you, please, what it is like here?"

Mimi thinks for a moment and says, "It's boring here. That is what it is like, it is boring."

She then looks at me and says, "May I ask you a personal question?"

"Sure," I say.

She wants to know if I have had a stroke, and tells me that I have the same symptoms as she does.

"Have you had a stroke?"

"No," I say. I explain again that I am writing about staying here, and that Aviston has a program for people to stay and feel a little of what it is like to live here.

Mimi says, "And you are staying here for a week."

"Yes."

"And after your week is done, you are going to stand up and walk out of here."

Saying yes to Mimi, yes, I will walk away, yes, I am fine, yes, it is a learning experience, yes, I am free to leave, yes, you are here and cannot leave, and, yes, we do not say it, but, yes, you will die here or at a place like here—this is the hardest lesson in empathy that I learned during my time at Aviston and the hardest challenge I had faced, much harder than any of the other challenges.

"I think you're lucky," Mimi says.

I ask her if she wants to write a poem together. I explain how I will ask her questions and write down her responses, and how what she shares with me will become the lines of her poem. I tell Mimi we will use as our model Wordsworth's poem "Daffodils." I ask her if she will perform the poem with me, explaining how call and response works. She laughs as we quietly perform the poem together.

And then my heart with pleasure fills
and dances with the daffodils.

I ask Mimi a series of questions, exploring spring through her senses. What does she think of when she hears the word *spring*? What does spring smell like to her? How does spring feel? What does spring sound like? Here is her poem:

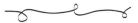

SPRING
—MIMI

I think of flowers, lilacs.
Spring smells like cut grass.
Spring feels warm.
Kids are playing baseball.
Yelling homerun!
I hear birds.
Red birds.

After we finish the poem, I thank Mimi and ask her if we might write another poem together and if she enjoyed the experience. "I liked it very much," she says.

I wheel away back to the dining area and Mimi starts her physical therapy. I take out my notebook and begin to write about my experience with Mimi. She is watching me, and when Leslie comes and sits with me, I know that Mimi thinks we are talking about her.

Later, it comes back to me through the grapevine that Mimi has been telling people I am a spy. She says that I am always writing down notes, and the staff should be really careful what they say around me. People tell her I am here as part of a program, but she does not buy it and is sure I must be a spy.

I do not see Mimi for the rest of the week. She does not come to the poetry reading I give for the residents on the last day. It is getting close to my time to leave for the airport, and I am saying good-byes. Leslie and I are having a final talk, checking in on how everything went. I feel so close to the people here.

I ask Leslie if she thinks it would be okay if I go back to Mimi's room, and she says she thinks it would be a good thing to do.

I wheel myself back there and Mimi looks up as I get to her doorway.

"May I come in and speak with you?" I ask.

"Yes," she says.

"I wanted to tell you thanks for writing the poem with me."

"Thank you," she says.

"I am always taking notes because I am trying to learn what it is like to live here. You have helped me learn that."

"You are not a spy?"

"No, I am not a spy."

"But I saw you talking to Leslie."

"Yes, Leslie is my friend and I do talk to her about my experience here."

"Did you tell her what I said about it being boring?"

"Yes, and Leslie wants to hear what you think. Is there anything you want me to tell Leslie for you?"

Mimi thinks for a while and says, "Yes, there should be more staff on this wing."

"Thank you, I will tell her. I have really enjoyed meeting you, Mimi."

"You are leaving now?"

"Yes."

"And you are going to get up and walk out of here?"

"Yes."

"You are so lucky."

Memory Arts Café and the Memory Arts Bistro
Memory Arts Café Day

The room was packed with more than 100 people, as Nan Blackshear, the liaison for the office of the Brooklyn Borough President, read the official proclamation:

> Whereas, it is a time-honored Brooklyn tradition to honor those extraordinary individuals . . .
>
> Whereas, all of Brooklyn joins as . . . the New York Memory Center gathers together alongside the Alzheimer's Poetry Project . . . on the momentous and auspicious occasion of the opening of New York State's first Memory Arts Café—a series of free art events tailored to those living with Alzheimer's disease and their caregivers.
>
> Whereas, on behalf of all Brooklynites, I salute the leadership of the New York Memory Center and the Alzheimer's Poetry Project. . . . I thank all those who have dedicated their lives to eliminating one of the leading causes of disability in the United States, which well help make Brooklyn and beyond better and healthier places to live, work, and raise a family.
>
> Now, therefore, I, Marty Markowitz, President of the Borough of Brooklyn, do hereby proclaim Wednesday, June 13th, 2012.
>
> *New York Memory Center*
> *Memory Arts Café Opening*
> *Celebration Day in Brooklyn, U.S.A.*

Christopher Nadeau, Executive Director of the New York Memory Center, had agreed to partner with the Alzheimer's Poetry Project to create a Memory Arts Café. He had done an excellent job of securing proclamations from

Markowitz, the City of New York Department on Aging, and New York City Mayor Michael Bloomberg. For me, a Brooklynite, it was Marty's stamp of approval that counted. We were also excited to receive funding for the project from the Alzheimer's Foundation of America.

After Nan had finished reading, I asked if she would help us create a proclamation, Alzheimer's Poetry Project style. She and I led the audience in a call and response chant:

> Whereas, the Memory Arts Café is a cool place, and we all gathered here today are cats and kittens, and in the words of the immortal Lord Buckley, "Hipsters, flipsters, and finger-poppin' daddies, and we are here to dig us some jazz.

> Whereas, our guest artists, Louise and Mark, are lovers of jazz, and they will lead us unto the creation of our own jazzy, jazz, jazz song.

> Whereas, Marty Markowitz is the hippest Borough President known to mankind, won't you join me in quoting from the immortal Jackie Gleason, in the sheep's wool of Ralph Kramden of "The Honeymooners" fame, life in Brooklyn, wait for it, ready here it comes . . . *How sweet it is! How sweet it is!* Yes, Goddess of the Brooklyn Bridge almighty, *How sweet it is!*

Creating a Memory Arts Café

With the Memory Arts Café in Brooklyn we wanted to provide a safe and welcoming environment where artists of all genres can collaborate to create and perform work with people living with Alzheimer's disease and related dementia, along with their family members. We hold our culminating event in partnership with the Brooklyn Museum.

We bring leading artists together at the Memory Arts Café to push forward the arts-in-healthcare movement. Building on the Alzheimer's Café movement in Europe, an idea pioneered by Dr. Bère Miesen, a clinical geriatric psychologist at the Specialist Research Center for Old-Age Psychiatry in the Netherlands, the Memory Arts Café expands that social model and places the creativity of people navigating cognitive impairment at the core of this innovative arts project.

The overarching goal of this project is to facilitate collaborative working practices among artists in the arts-in-healthcare field and the Alzheimer's Poetry Project. Our goal is to help people living with dementia and their family members explore their creativity and to show, through evidence-based research, that a life that includes creativity leads to an increased quality of life. The objective is to create a replicable curriculum based on the shared elements of interactive arts projects for people living with dementia.

Brief History of Alzheimer's Café, or Memory Cafés

- In 1997, Dr. Bère Miesen launched the first café in Holland.

- In 2000, the idea spread to the United Kingdom with the launch of its first café, largely through the work of Kandy Redwood, a Carers Support Worker at Hampshire County Council in England.

- In 2008, Dr. Jytte Lokvig, an Alzheimer's activist and author of *The Alzheimer's Creativity Project*, among other books, introduced the first Alzheimer's Café to the United States in Santa Fe, New Mexico.

Dr. Miesen, in his opening address for the first Alzheimer's Café United Kingdom national conference, described the concept of an Alzheimer's café:

> An Alzheimer Café is intended to be a real café. In other words, you don't have to book a place before going there, you can come and go as you please; there's food and drink available there, you can listen to some music, talk about what you're going through, you can always find a listening ear, and you can remain anonymous, if that's what you want to do.

In formal terms, the Alzheimer's Café concept can be described as a low-threshold group intervention for anyone affected by dementia, integrating all the benefits of an ordinary café. And this holds true in terms of psychological-education, information, and therapeutic contact with professionals and people in the same situation.

I personally find the Alzheimer's Café to be a sort of ritual for ridding oneself of fear and emotional separation and for maintaining a long-term resistance against what is happening.

How a Memory Arts Café Is Structured

Using the Brooklyn Memory Arts Café as a model, a typical gathering is structured as follows:

- For the first 30 minutes the group socializes over snacks and drinks. We take the role of host seriously and make sure people are introduced to each other and to the guest artist.

- As the host of an event, I interview the guest artist for about 10 minutes in front of the audience (not for too long, but enough time for the group to get to know the person). I ask questions such as how the person got started and describe a favorite or rewarding moment as an artist. I might ask the artist to explain a little of his or her work or, if the guest artist is a musician, to talk about why he or she chose that instrument and how it works. The audience is encouraged to ask questions as well.

- To end the interview I ask the artist to perform a short piece in the 3-to-5-minute range, so the audience can get a sense of his or her work. As a poet, I often work with the guest artist to combine a duet with dance and poetry or music and poetry.

- During the next 15 minutes, the guest artist creates a new work with the audience. For example, we had Heidi Latsky, a choreographer who works with disabled communities, create a dance with us. For another gathering, the jazz singer Louise Rogers and pianist Mark Kross created a blues piece about Brooklyn.

- Once we have created the new work, we perform the piece with the audience. The key to the Memory Arts Café is that the performances are participatory. Everybody joins in and works together.

While there is nothing wrong with a traditional style concert where you listen to a professional performance, including the audience in the creation and performance of the new work honors them as people who remain creative, even while navigating memory loss. This is often where the family members get to see a side of their loved one that is heartening. The person is laughing, singing, and dancing. While the participatory performance is happening, you might even feel that there is no dementia in the room.

Christopher Nadeau, Executive Director, and Josephine Brown, Program Director, of the New York Memory Center and co-producers of the Memory Arts Café, talk about the project's impact:

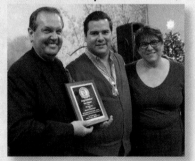

(Josephine) The Memory Arts Café lets us show participants how to communicate through the arts, through reading a poem, doing a dance, attending the Memory Arts Café. It makes it possible to meet people who are going through the same thing. Support groups are wonderful, but this is the ultimate support group. The families are communicating with each other. One caregiver has an appointment and can't get a home attendant and she has other caregivers to call and say, "Can I drop my mom off and have you help with her?" It's paid back, and they are sharing the care.

Josephine Brown, Christopher Nadeau, and Gary Glazner

They are opening new doors on how to help each other. They are forming networks of support. They are learning how to work with their loved ones better, communicate with them better. They talk to each other about how they handle problems, without being stressed out so much. It's amazing. It's incredible the way they have come together. We have families that didn't know each other, but who are coming to the Memory Arts Café. And now they are going to each other's house for tea and planning barbecues for the staff to thank them for bringing them together.

It's visual. They are seeing how to use art to communicate with their loved one. Whether it's poetry, music, dance, or a movie, they can share the experience together, and it is bringing families together as a bigger community.

(Christopher) The Memory Arts Café is not only destigmatizing the disease, it's opening the doorway for therapeutic communication. Before that, let's say every six months, we do a seminar on therapeutic communication. You can reinforce the lessons over and over again, but unless the person with dementia sees on a deep personal level what that means, that you enter their world, and that means that you can't communicate with them on the same basis that you did before.

Once you engage in the creative arts and see the happiness you share together, that opens a doorway to how to be more therapeutic in the home setting. What we would teach in educational seminars we are now showing in the Memory Arts Café without even having to talk about it directly. Without having to reinforce the principles of therapeutic communication, it's now the family saying, "I see, I understand, I can work with my Mom in a different way. We are having fun doing this and this is a great way to communicate."

The Memory Arts Bistro

One of the absolute blasts of working in the dementia arts community is the people you get to meet. I met Michelle Dionisio, President and CEO of Benevilla, at the America Society on Aging Conference in Chicago in 2013. A nonprofit human services agency, Benevilla assists people in remaining independent and in their own homes for as long as possible. After a talk I gave in which I described starting the Memory Arts Café with my partners at the New York Memory Center, Michelle spoke with me about the Benevilla community in Surprise, Arizona, and how they had a perfect venue for a café, only they were going to tap into their chef's expertise and make it a Memory Arts Bistro!

I was thrilled when she said the magic words, "What would it take to get you to come out and be our first guest artist?" That was how I found myself on a beautiful fall day in Arizona dancing to the groove of percussionist Gene Jones as Michelle led the audience in some of the moves from their Zoomba Alzheimer's Class.

Memory Arts Bistro

Michelle Dionisio, President and CEO of Benevilla in Arizona, discusses the mission of Benevilla and how their Memory Arts Bistro furthers the goals of the community:

Benevilla is a health and human services organization that was formed 32 years ago by the residents in Sun City, Arizona, who wanted to live with independence and dignity and to age gracefully in the community. Today, Benevilla has expanded their mission beyond the elderly, to families and children of the northwest valley, which has 600,000 residents. The mission is to enhance the experience of life for people of all ages and we accomplish this through engaging community residents by providing direct human and health services, offering opportunities in volunteer work, and celebrating the assets of our community, such as the arts, intergenerational programs, and lifelong learning.

We organized the Memory Arts Bistro by bringing together Benevilla staff leaders, community volunteers and the West Valley Arts Council. At the beginning we created a mission statement, which read: "The purpose of the Memory Arts Bistro is to provide a welcoming social and arts environment . . . for individuals with memory loss and their family and/or caregivers that will provide opportunities to explore their creativity, offer support and socialization."

As we planned the Memory Arts Bistro, we knew it would require financial support in order to provide this free social and interactive arts program. We wanted to have quality artists, musicians, and art supplies available and offer free catered food (appetizers and refreshments) to ensure its success. Both Benevilla and the West Valley Arts Council have had experience with soliciting local business and corporate sponsors for other fundraising events. I believe the importance of getting sponsors helps to provide sustainability for the project, gets the word out to the greater community about this wonderful program, and gives sponsors great exposure to potential customers.

The Memory Arts Bistro furthers our goals to serve area residents with quality, meaningful art experiences to help improve their health and well-being and give support and social opportunities to their caregivers in an accepting, supportive environment.

I believe the ability to provide quality interactive arts programs for area residents will truly improve their quality of life and ability to remain living at home in the community.

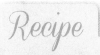

CONEY ISLAND AQUARIUM JELLYFISH JELLY JAM

INGREDIENTS:

1 under the brine poem by Walt Whitman
1 recording of "Under the Boardwalk"
1 player (MP3, iPad, iPod, or smartphone will do, or go old school and bring a boom box with a CD player)
1 set of portable speakers

INSTRUCTIONS:

One of my favorite Memory Arts Café field trips was to visit the New York Aquarium at Coney Island. Below is the poem we created on the field trip. We were inspired by the "*Jellyfish*-Alien Stingers" exhibit and created the poem by asking the participants to describe the jellyfish. We sang "Under the Boardwalk" and recited poems about the ocean, including Walt Whitman's "The World Below the Brine," with its wonderful line,

> "...Different colors, pale gray and green, purple, white,
> and gold, the play of light through the water..."

(To see a performance of the poem, go to http://www.youtube.com/user/alzpoetry, click on Videos, and then scroll until you find "Jellyfish.")

I learned the trick of using an iPad with portable speakers to bring music to workshops from Maria Genné of Kairos Alive! Dance Theater. She and her group use the recording to great effect to enhance their dance workshops. I love it for adding a little spice with a well-known song, and for a person like me, who has trouble holding a melody, it is invaluable.

The group only had to hear the opening notes of "Under the Boardwalk" and immediately began singing along with gusto. We had a lot of fun being playful with the low bass coming in on the "Under the Boardwalk, BOARDWALK! BOARDWALK!!

We drew crowds of families who joined in with the singing and helped out by giving responses to our questions when we began to create our

continued

poem. The aquarium program director had a big smile when one little boy answered the question "What do you think of when you think of Jellyfish?" with "Run for your life! I hope they don't sting me." He had everyone laughing. Another highlight was Ola offering unprompted, "Oh, I see a jellyfish. How I wish they were on a dish, because I'm hungry!"

Jellyfish

Jelly, jelly, cha, cha, cha . . .

They are just the cutest little things
I have ever seen.

Stinging!
Run for your life!
I hope they don't sting me.

Peanut butter and jellyfish!

A delicate balance.
A delicate dance.
Wearing our delicate jellyfish pants.

They are stingy and stringy and slimy.
They are fast.
They are beautiful.

Oh, I see a jellyfish.
How I wish they were on a dish,
Because I'm hungry!

They look like clouds floating in the water.
Tranquility.
Liquid buttons.

continued

THE BATH

HOLLY J. HUGHES

The tub fills inch by inch,
as I kneel beside it, trail my fingers
in the bright braid of water.
Mom perches on the toilet seat,
entranced by the ritual until
she realizes the bath's for her.
Oh no, she says, drawing her
three layers of shirts to her chest,
crossing her arms and legs.
Oh no, I couldn't, she repeats,
brow furrowing, that look I now
recognize like an approaching squall.
I abandon reason, the hygiene argument,
promise a Hershey's bar, if she will just,
please, take off her clothes. Oh no,
she repeats, her voice rising.
Meanwhile, the water is cooling.
I strip off my clothes, step into it,
let the warm water take me
completely, slipping down until
only my face shines up, a moon mask.
Mom stays with me, interested now
in this turn of events. I sit up.
Will you wash my back, Mom?
So much gone, but let this
still be there. She bends over
to dip the washcloth in the still
warm water, squeezes it,
lets it dribble down my back,
leans over to rub the butter pat
of soap, swiping each armpit,
then rinses off the suds with long
practiced strokes. I turn around
to thank her, catch her smiling,
lips pursed, humming,
still a mother with a daughter
whose back needs washing.

(From Beyond Forgetting: Poetry and Prose about Alzheimer's Disease, edited by Holly J. Hughes [2009, Kent State University Press, used by permission])

Dementia-Friendly Communities

I filled a bucket full of snow and carried it around the room offering it up to people who were gathered to recite and create poems. They touched the snow and laughed. Some tasted it and remarked on the pureness of Wisconsin snow. Others said it was too cold for them, and no thanks. The group talked about building snowmen and sang parts of a song about a fellow named Frosty.

It was a cold day in February and my first experience working on a dementia-friendly community project as part of the Fox Valley Memory Project in Appleton, Wisconsin. As I prepared to start the poetry session, I took a seat next to a woman who had been quiet during the snow sharing. I sat the bucket down at her feet and asked if she would take care of it. She smiled and moved it closer to her. Throughout the session she would touch the snow and smile and took seriously her role as snow guardian or, yes, snow angel.

What Is a Dementia-Friendly Community?

First, a huge shout out to Norms McNamara and the Torbay Dementia Action Alliance in Torbay, England, who are a major proponent and organizer of the movement to create dementia-friendly communities.

As part of the Fox Valley Memory Project, one of the first in the United States and launched in 2013, persons with memory loss expressed their wishes for a community, including

- Has somewhere you can go to stimulate your mind and ask questions

- Has friends I can just be with and people who understand

- Allows people in nursing homes to be taken out, even just for a ride

- Offers more things I can do in the community, like Memory Cafés

The Alzheimer's Poetry Project worked with the Fox Valley Memory Project in providing outreach to the community using the arts as a communication tool. We facilitated in-depth training over a 3-month period for 15 healthcare workers from 5 assisted living centers. We held a culminating poetry party and infused the Fox Valley Memory Project's first field trip with poetry. Fifty-five people took part in the field trip, during which we visited a chocolate factory, shared a wonderful lunch, and took a river cruise. We performed the poem we created together on the bus ride home. Here is the poem we created on the field trip.

FIRST EVER! WORLD PREMIER! INAUGURAL FOX RIVER & CHOCOLATE TASTING EXTRAVAGANZA POEM!

(The 55 poets of the Fox Valley Memory Project, with poet Gary Glazner and organizers John and Susan McFadden and Betty Lefebvre-Hill, wrote this poem on July 24th, 2013. These words set forth here commemorate the initial Fox Valley Memory Project field trip to Seroogy's Homemade Chocolates, the River Room Restaurant, and a cruise on the Fox River. Which, by the way, did you know the river flows north?)

When I think of today, I think of fellowship,
Getting together to go to the river.

On the subject of chocolate:
I ate the whole piece!
Very smooth, sweet and just about perfect.
It bloomed in my mouth.
The taste of chocolate is friendly.

The coffee is good and hot.
Do you like it creamy?

Oooooooooo that chocolate was good.
The melt aways caused us to buy meltaways.
How would I describe the chocolate?
Uuuuuuum, uuuuuuum smooooth stuff!

On the subject of lunch:
Chicken, chicken, fish, chicken, chicken, fish.
Fabulous, tasty, excellent!
How would I describe the fish? Swimmingly!

On the subject of the river:
It's great, the first time I have had a river ride.

Lots of history.
We were raised a little way from here.
I love the white pelicans.
The lazy ones who don't want to fly all
the way to Canada.

A wonderful bird is the pelican,
His bill will hold more than his belican.
He can take in his beak
Food enough for a week,
But I'm damned if I see how the helican.

I love the water.
I love being out on a beautiful day.
Letting the boat rock me to sleep.

I like to go on the water but I don't want to be in the water.

There are lots of things I love about today.
What do I like about today?
Being out in the fresh air, the sunlight and the chocolate.

Enjoying the view on a perfect day.
I did not realize there was so much on the river.

I love seeing my mom out and enjoying herself
The smile on her face.

I like seeing bridges going up.
Seeing this part of the river.

There is nothing like being on the water.
I love the calming effect.
Let someone else do the driving.

A Place at the Table for Dementia Arts

APP is committed to fostering similar partnerships through outreach and staff trainings, with the goal of incorporating the arts in dementia care. Our most recent partnership is with the state of New Mexico. In October 2013, the state released the New Mexico State Plan for Alzheimer's Disease and Related Dementias.

The Letter of Introduction in part reads:

> The prevalence of Alzheimer's disease and related dementias is an issue that will soon reach monumental proportions in New Mexico and the nation. Addressing this issue will require a major commitment from a host of individuals, businesses, government agencies and healthcare providers, and a new and vibrant level of collaboration among all those partners.

For me, while incredibly thoughtful and detailed, the plan is notable in that it does not include any specific goal of incorporating the arts in dementia care. Considering the scope of care and education they want to facilitate, dementia arts seemed a natural fit to help them accomplish their goals.

As a person dedicated to dementia arts, and given the fact that the Alzheimer's Poetry Project was started in New Mexico, I knew I had to act.

My first step was to write to the office of the Governor of New Mexico, Susan Martinez, and ask for a meeting to discuss ways that the Alzheimer's Poetry Project could support the plan. James William Ross, Cabinet Director, Office of the Governor, and Miles Copeland, Deputy Director, New Mexico Department on Aging, agreed to meet with us.

Next, I identified key elements of the plan for which APP could support the efforts of the plan stakeholders.

Then I gathered a team to support me at the meeting: Tom Leech, Curator and Director of the Palace Press at New Mexico History Museum; Michelle Otero, the APP Spanish Language Director; Edie Song, the Creator of Snow Poems; Joan Logghe, President of New Mexico Literary Arts and Valerie Martinez, Director of Little Globe. Both Logghe and Martinez are past poet laureates of Santa Fe.

The end result of the meeting is that we are planning to hold the Dementia Arts Training at the New Mexico History Museum and launch the first dementia-friendly community in New Mexico in 2014.

Below are the goals of the New Mexico plan and suggestions for how APP and our partners can infuse the arts in support of each.

Goal 1. Develop an adequate network structure.

- Identify current resources and enhance communication and collaboration between these resources in a manner that maximizes their state impact in all areas of the state plan, including: meeting caregiver needs; elevating quality of care; broadening public awareness of dementia and available resources; matching healthcare system capacity to consumer need; and increasing research effectiveness.

APP contribution and support:

- Communicate and collaborate with other groups on how best to meet caregiver needs, elevate quality of care, and increase public awareness of resources.

- Host dementia arts conference and training for caregivers, healthcare professionals, museum staff, teaching artists, and the interested general public.

- Work in partnership with those groups implementing the New Mexico State Plan for Alzheimer's Disease and Related Dementias on a pilot project to create a dementia-friendly community in Los Cruces. This would be based on APP's partnership in the spring of 2013 with the Fox Valley Memory Project. This pilot project would then be used as a blueprint for other communities in New Mexico.

Goal 2. Expand public awareness and dementia resource connections:

- Identify and encourage coordination, collaboration, and inter-entity communication with public and private, local, state, and federal entities to advance Alzheimer's readiness and dementia-capable systems.

- Conduct a public awareness campaign, particularly to address the diverse ethnic, cultural, linguistic, and literacy differences in the state.

- Expand access to culturally appropriate resources and supports for family caregivers and all populations and entities that care for and treat individuals with Alzheimer's disease and related dementias.

APP contribution and support:

- Communicate and collaborate with other groups on APP programming and training, including Spanish-language programming.

Goal 3. Support and empower unpaid caregivers:

- Expand evidence-based caregiver training in a manner that is effective across New Mexico cultures and locations.

- Engage caregivers in culture training in English and Spanish on the use of oral histories to create poems and stories with their loved ones.

Goal 4: Expand research opportunities in New Mexico:

- Identify and expand existing data sources and develop new data sources; determine how best to ensure analysis and use of data.

- Provide New Mexico Alzheimer's Plan partners current research on dementia arts.

Goal 5: Support education and training for a dementia-competent workforce:

- Expand education and training through collaborations between New Mexico state universities, branch colleges, community and technical colleges, and private institutions.

- Provide education and training to New Mexico businesses to help them become dementia friendly.

In conclusion, APP is thrilled to be providing support to the state of New Mexico in implementing its Plan for Alzheimer's Disease and Related Dementias. We see this partnership as a blueprint for working with others to help create dementia-friendly communities across the country and abroad.

Building Community
On Passing the Smile as Metaphor for Passing on the Legacy

Elders Share the Arts

I like to think of the improvisation game "pass the smile" when I think of Elders Share the Arts (ESTA), which was founded by Susan Perlstein. ESTA is one of the pioneers in the field of "creative aging," which focuses on the direct and beneficial impact of creative engagement on the overall physical, mental, and emotional health of older adults. They have worked with older adults in community-based sites throughout New York City to empower them in finding and giving creative voice to their life stories and experiences. The image of passing a smile from one person to the next feels like what Susan has done with Jennie Smith-Peers, currently the executive director of ESTA.

In 2001, ESTA was selected to be one of four participating sites nationwide in the groundbreaking research study "Creativity and Aging," conducted by Dr. Gene Cohen, Director of the Institute on Health, Humanities, and Aging at The George Washington University. (See http://arts.gov/sites/default/files/CnA-Rep4-30-06.pdf) Published in 2006 and the first longitudinal study of its kind, Dr. Cohen's research found a direct link between creative expression and healthy aging. Cohen once said that art "is like chocolate for the brain." He believes that creativity in older adults can flourish with greater depth and richness given the vast knowledge and experiences that inform their creative efforts. This belief inspires and continues to be reflected in each of ESTA's programs.

Continuing with the metaphor of passing the smile as passing on legacy, Gene Cohen passed on his love of creative aging to ESTA and in founding the National Center for Creative Aging (NCCA) with Susan Perlstein and Gay Hannah.

National Center for Creative Aging

Another important person in my life is Dr. Gay Hanna, Executive Director of National Center for Creative Aging (NCCA). I am proud to have recently joined the board of the NCCA. They are the leading advocacy group for creative aging and are really developing and pushing the field forward with initiatives such as their Teaching Artists Training, Creative Aging Directory, and Communities of Practice, among many other wonderful projects and resources. You may read more about their programs at http://www.creativeaging.org/.

I Never Told Anybody

The poet Kenneth Koch has also passed on his knowledge of creative aging through his book, *I Never Told Anybody: Teaching Poetry Writing to Old People* (1977). The idea of creating poetry by giving people writing prompts and then taking dictation directly informs the APP's method of creating poems by asking open-ended questions and writing down the participants' responses to form the lines of the poem.

Koch writes,

> …I taught poetry writing at the American Nursing Home in New York City on the Lower East Side, at Avenue B and 5th Street. I had about twenty-five students, and we met sixteen times, usually on Wednesday mornings for about an hour. The students were all incapacitated in some way, by illness or old age. Most were in their seventies, eighties, and nineties. Most were from the working class and had a limited education. They had worked as dry cleaners, messengers, short-order cooks, domestic servants. A few had worked in offices, and one had been an actress. The nursing home gave them safety and care and a few activities, and sometimes a trip to a show or museum. They did little or no reading or writing. They had not written poetry prior to my teaching the workshop. (p. 3)

For me Koch is a major touchstone in working with people living with dementia. So 35 years later, when I led an intergenerational program with the young women of the Lower East Side Girls Club and the elders at Cabrini Center for Nursing & Rehabilitation Center, something about the location rang a bell. I went back to Koch's detailed description, which included the cross streets for the American Nursing Home and, yes, it was the same address. Cabrini had leased the same Lower East Side site at 542 E. 5th Street at Avenue B. We had come full circle and, as if we are passing the smile, we were in the building Koch had worked in all those years ago. My feel for his passing on his legacy deepened when I read this passage at the end of *I Never Told Anybody*:

> . . . No matter where we had stopped, it would have been in the middle. I thought it would be sad and wasteful if the workshop ended, so I had asked other poets to come to a few classes, hoping that one of them would like to continue it. David Lehman did, and gave classes on through most of the summer. . . . The poems which follow from David Lehman's class . . . will, I hope, suggest that it is not only with one particular teacher that old and ill people can be helped to write so well, nor only in one place. (p. 231)

There it is, a call from Koch to continue the work, to pass the smile. At our first session with the Girls Club, one of the young women had chosen Sonnet 18 by Shakespeare as her poem to present. As she started in with the famous opening line, "Shall I compare thee to a summer's day," we heard a deep voice join in with her, amazed the young woman stopped reading as a distinguished older gentleman recited the poem by heart. We all cheered as he passed on his love of Shakespeare and Shakespeare passed on his pledge that

As long as men can breath or eyes can see
So long lives this and this gives life to thee.

As the poem is more than 400 years, it seems that Shakespeare's boast just might be true, and that the love in the poem lives on to be passed on again and again.

One of the earliest passages I have found that deals with old age is this famous monologue from Shakespeare's "As You Like It."

All the World's a Stage

All the world's a stage,
And all the men and women merely players;
They have their exits and their entrances,
And one man in his time plays many parts,
His acts being seven ages. At first, the infant,
Mewling and puking in the nurse's arms.
Then the whining schoolboy, with his satchel
And shining morning face, creeping like snail
Unwillingly to school. And then the lover,
Sighing like furnace, with a woeful ballad
Made to his mistress' eyebrow. Then a soldier,
Full of strange oaths and bearded like the pard,
Jealous in honor, sudden and quick in quarrel,
Seeking the bubble reputation
Even in the cannon's mouth. And then the justice,
In fair round belly with good capon lined,

With eyes severe and beard of formal cut,
Full of wise saws and modern instances;
And so he plays his part. The sixth age shifts
Into the lean and slippered pantaloon,
With spectacles on nose and pouch on side;
His youthful hose, well saved, a world too wide
For his shrunk shank, and his big manly voice,
Turning again toward childish treble, pipes
And whistles in his sound. Last scene of all,
That ends this strange eventful history,
Is second childishness and mere oblivion,
Sans teeth, sans eyes, sans taste, sans everything.

Poetry Slam

My first experience in building community around poetry was in working with the Poetry Slam. For more than 10 years, from 1990 to 2002, I worked on a daily basis to help the Poetry Slam grow. I served on the original board when the movement shifted from being grassroots to formalizing as a non-profit. I edited one of the first books to document the movement, *Poetry Slam: The Competitive Art of Performance Poetry* (2000). I topped off my work with the Poetry Slam in 2001, when I organized the Slam America tour. The tour was 30 readings in 30 cities in 30 days, and our official slogan was "One Million Miles of Poetry."

My life changed when I met poet Marc Smith, who is credited with inventing the poetry slam at the Get Me High Lounge in Chicago in 1984. In July 1986, the slam moved to its permanent home, the Green Mill Jazz Club. In 1990, working with Marc Smith, I produced the first National Poetry Slam in Fort Mason, San Francisco, involving a team from Chicago and San Francisco, as well as an individual poet from New York City. The event took place as part of the National Poetry Association's International Poetry Festival, which was organized by poets Jack Mueller and Herman Berlandt. As of 2013, the National Poetry Slam has grown and currently features 80 certified teams each year, culminating in 5 days of competition.

Overseeing the National Poetry Slam annual event was an amazing training opportunity to learn how to build community around poetry, and those are lessons I use everyday in building the Alzheimer's Poetry Project.

Marc has a poem, "Pull the Next One Up," that perfectly embodies the idea of building community around poetry or art and always makes me smile when I hear it. To give you a sense and little taste of Marc's work, here are the opening and closing lines:

When you get to the top of the mountain
Pull the next one up.
Then there'll be two of you
Roped together at the waist
Tired and proud, knowing the mountain,
Knowing the human force it took
To bring both of you there . . .

. . . That the only courage there is is
To pull the next man up
Pull the next woman up
Pull the next up

Up

Up.

So pull the next one up, and pass the smile!

Margery Pabst and the Pabst Charitable Foundation for the Arts

My life changed again when I met Margery Pabst. Out of all of the philanthropists I have worked with, Margery is the most interested in meeting with you, helping you think through what you are really trying to accomplish with a project, and challenging you to think big.

In 2012, Margery and I worked together to do community-wide training in APP's methods and techniques in her town of Winter Park, Florida. Since then we have taken what we learned there and adapted it to community-wide projects in Sheboygan and Appleton, Wisconsin. Much of what we learned centered around working with the various assisted living and adult day centers as well as their staff, who we trained to empower them to take ownership of using poetry to improve the quality of life of people living with memory loss.

These efforts have resulted in adding more training sessions and deepening the training with techniques you have read about throughout this book. One idea that has really taken root is to have the lead organization host a culminating event to celebrate the project. The flyer that follows is from the culminating event we held in Sheboygan, which was organized by The Gathering Place and is now in its second year.

creativity
is
ageless

Exploring Art with Alzheimer's

Tuesday, May 22, 2012
5:00 – 7:00 p.m.

Location: Breaking Bread Banquet Hall
6451 S. Business Dr., Sheboygan
Light hors d'ourves and cash bar

Explore the creative writing and art created by people with memory loss

Libby's House, Sheboygan Senior Community and
The Gathering Place proudly present an evening
of Arts, created by their residents. Gary Glazner,
international speaker and director of the
Alzheimer Poetry Project will showcase the
creative stories written by the residents.

Partially funded by Wisconsin Arts Board and Helen Bader Foundation.

**The art will be on display
at the following locations
prior to the art auction:**

Mead Public Library
Community Bank – Business Drive
Edward Jones – Brian Beeck, Sheboygan Falls
Bemis Bath Shoppe
Richardson Emporium
Sheboygan Falls Library
Kohler Credit Union – Kohler
Breaking Bread
Wilson Mutual Insurance
Tri Cor Insurance – Plymouth

1st annual
Artist Challenge and Auction
to benefit

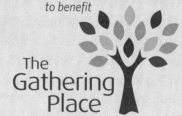

The
Gathering
Place

A sincere thank you to our corporate sponsors: Wilson Mutual Insurance and Breaking Bread

If you are reading this and thinking we would love to host a community-wide Alzheimer's Poetry Project training in our town, please know we are actively looking for opportunities and partners to work with. Feel free to contact us at gary@alzpoetry.org.

So let's pass the smile; share the arts; tell what you have never told anybody; pull the next one up; challenge each other to think big; seed the field and advocate for change; and eat a heart-shaped box of sweet treats labeled, "Art is like chocolate for the brain." Onward!

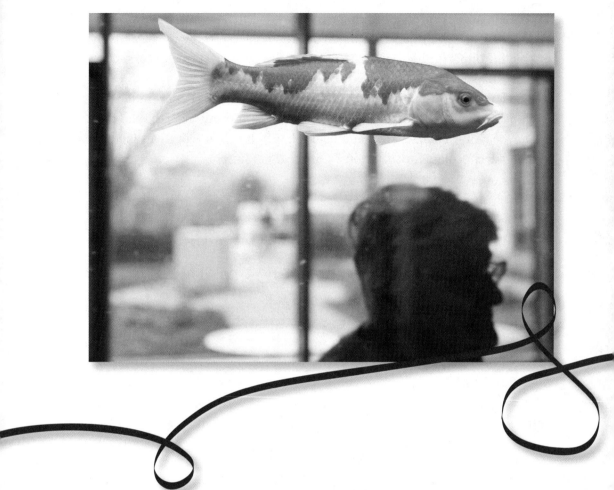

BIOLOGY
OF POETRY

Biology of Poetry

My first science experience was in grade school when I participated in the much-loved experiment of growing bean plants in a dark closet and a sunny spot to compare the growth of the plants. Can you guess which grew better? For this section we shift from using recipes to the language of a science fair to describe a research project that the Alzheimer's Poetry Project has embarked on with the Dementia Arts Research Ensemble. The project is being funded by the Alzheimer's Foundation of America to investigate the effectiveness of using poetry and other art forms in creating rich stimuli to improve the quality of life of people living with Alzheimer's disease and related dementia.

Psychobiology

I trace my personal history and interest in the biology of poetry to a ball of spit that would form on my professor's lip as he lectured. He seemed oblivious to the glob, dangling and defying gravity as he excitedly introduced us to synapses, axons, neurotransmitters, brain structures such as the amygdala and hippocampus, and what in 1980 was the new discipline of psychobiology. That was also the year I began writing and studying poetry.

Merriam-Webster defines *psychobiology* as, "the study of mental functioning and behavior in relation to other biological processes." The professor, with his shaggy beard and thick glasses, was the epitome of the absent-minded scientist. However, he was so acutely aware of human behavior that it seemed more likely his habit of spit balls was some bizarre experiment on his part to focus our attention. You could not look away; would the ball drop or not? He was a fascinating lecturer and made the concept of understanding our behavior and the brain come alive.

Thirty years later, I use the knowledge gained in that class on a daily basis in trying to understand the brains of people living with memory loss. Since I began using poetry with people living with dementia, I have often thought back to that class and see a strong connection between my fascination with that early exposure to psychobiology and my desire to explore poetry in a healthcare setting.

What was the biological basis for the response I was seeing in those I read classic poems to? I was finding that people with mid- to late-stage Alzheimer's disease, who could not recall if they had just drunk a glass of juice or remember the face of a friend or family member, could remember lines and words from poems. This has played out many times in many sessions and it always feels as if the poem were a switch that had turned the person on again.

Reverse Engineering the Muse

The poet Jane Hirshfield in her essay, "Poetry as Vessel of Remembrance," from her book, *Nine Gates: Entering the Mind of Poetry*, argues that the structure of our minds developed around the use of rhymed, rhythmic, beautifully shaped information, or poetry, as a memory tool. To think of how the Greeks thought of muses as a clue to the power of poetry and how poetry was the first memory tool is brilliant.

Hirschfield writes:

> The story of poetry has many beginnings. One is in Mnemosyne—Remembrance—earliest-born of the Greek Goddesses, mother of the muses and so also of the poem....

> To see how the requirements of memorability created poetry, we need first to imagine the nature of language and knowledge in a purely oral world. As a number of scholars have pointed out, before literacy, sound, not sight, is the sense-realm in which words exist....

> For words themselves are vessels of consciousness, but before the coming of letters placed into clay tablet, papyrus, or book, verbal thought could live only in the fragile containers of inner contemplation and spoken language. Verse, at its most fundamental, is language put into the forms of remembrance. The earliest vessel for holding consciousness that has lasted, poetry is the progenitor of all the technologies of memory to come.

This is reverse muse, or looking for explanations of the success in using poetry with people living with dementia. I know poetry works because I see it in the faces of those I work with; I hear it in their voices. One sees how animated the group becomes after an hour of performing and creating poems.

Homer as Homeboy

Expanding from Hirshfield's Greek example, we have the tradition of African Griots, who over centuries have kept their village history in epic poems. In the connection between Griots and modern-day hip-hop, we see the improvisational form of rapping or free-styling that has a strong oral-poetry component. Hip-hop tells the stories of the African-American community and is a modern example of how poetry functions as Hirshfield imagines it, in pre-history times and central to the hip-hop culture of today.

Because of the influence of hip-hop, more people today are inspired to write rhyming, rhythmic verse than at anytime in the history of the world. One may argue the merit of the work as poetry, but it would be hard to exclude hip-hop using any common definition of poetry. Many of the kids in the classrooms I have taught in as a poet have been intensely interested in hip-hop. They may be our strongest examples of the attraction of our brains to using rhyme and rhythm.

Cowboy Poets

With their annual festivals of more than 10,000 people in Elko, Nevada, and Lubbock, Texas, Cowboy Poetry Gatherings may be the most popular poetry events in the United States. Cowboy poets, with their life-style and throwback to rhymed and rhythmic couplets as a way to maintain the stories of the ranching communities, are more examples of what Hirschfield sees as muses and of poetry playing an "absolutely central place in human life."

Test Our Working Hypothesis by Doing an Experiment

Working Hypothesis

Merriam-Webster defines *working hypothesis* as "a hypothesis adopted as a guide to experiment or investigate or as a basis of action." Our working hypothesis is the following:

If there is a relationship between a person living with memory loss expressing creativity while participating in the recitation and creation of poetry and positive emotional responses, then there is an indication of an increased quality of life.

Step A: Do Background Research

Background Research

The question running through my mind is how the brain of a person living with Alzheimer's disease and related dementia processes and experiences poetry? While we know a lot about the brain and are making breakthroughs in understanding Alzheimer's disease, scientists have still not discovered a cause or cure. As an artist, the place where our knowledge ends and theories start is an exciting place to be.

Central to my understanding of how poetry functions is a concept furthered by the poet Jane Hirshfield, that before written language was developed humans used poetry as a tool to record their history. She points to the Greek muse of memory, Mnemosyne, and connects this idea to Homer, who used the epic oral poems "The Odyssey" and "The Iliad" to tell the history of the Greeks.

Another key component that shaped my thinking about poetry was a study done in 2004 in Austria and Germany that showed that reciting poetry has an aerobic benefit and can thereby reduce stress indicators.

I was also thrilled to hear of a study from 2006 called the "Shakespeared Brain," which showed that Shakespearean language excites positive brain activity. Professor Philip Davis of the University of Liverpool monitored 20 participants as selected lines from Shakespeare's plays were read to them. Using Functional Magnetic Resonance Imaging, or fMRI, which measures brain activity by detecting associated changes in blood flow, Davis tested for a dramatic response in the language centers of the brain to a certain grammatical technique used by Shakespeare called functional shift (when one part of speech shifts to another, in this case where a noun shifts to a verb). Davis gives the example of the line "he godded me" from Shakespeare's tragedy *Coriolanus*, which is an unusual way of saying "he treated me like a god." The noun *God* shifts to the verb *godded*.

Dr. Davis's study highlights the following areas of interest:

- Heightened use of language increases synaptic activity in the language centers of the brain.

- Poetry, with its use of image, metaphor, and simile, is heightened use of language at its best.

This study helped to focus my thinking of how poetry might function on a biological level. The anecdotal responses of increased social engagement, brightening of affect, and being more present and more focused in our poetry sessions are partially based on poetry exciting the brain.

The work of Dr. Eric Kandel further encourages our look at how poetry might function on a neurological level and gives a basis to better understand the Shakespeared Brain. Dr. Kandel won the Nobel Prize in Physiology or Medicine in 2000 for showing how neurotransmitters create short- and long-term memory. In his books *In Search of Memory* and *The Age of Insight: The Quest to Understand the Unconscious in Art, Mind, and Brain, from Vienna 1900 to the Present*, he lays out his theories for the lay person.

Dr. Kandel's work highlights the following area of interest:

- When a person hears a poem that they learned as a child, the recitation of the words causes the firing of the synapses in the brain that are involved in the recall of that long-term memory.

This may explain the wonderful occurrence of someone living with memory loss finishing a line of poetry after hearing the first part, or of their knowing the end rhyme. For instance, I have worked with many people who, after hearing me recite "Quoth the raven . . . " from Edgar Allen Poe's "The Raven," will call out "Nevermore."

In linking these areas of thought, I seek to give a framework of evidence to support the robust response to poetry I have seen in thousands of people navigating cognitive impairment.

Reciting Poetry for Stress Reduction

Like many poets, I read with interest articles on the 2004 study, "Oscillations of Heart Rate and Respiration Synchronize during Poetry Recitation," when it first published. It was only later in tracking down the full paper and reading it in detail that I learned the researchers had used the technique of call and response in leading the participants in reciting poetry. (http://ajpheart. physiology.org/content/287/2/H579)

While the study received a great deal of press, it is less known that the researchers used call and response in combination with movement to regulate the subjects' breathing: "The subject listened to the text recited by the therapist without lifting the arms (but continued walking) and subsequently repeated it in the therapist's fashion."

The scientists concluded that, "In our own investigations on cardiovascular and cardiorespiratory regulation during and after recitation of poetry, we were led by the observation of therapists that creative arts greatly influence well-being in humans by various means."

The study highlights the following areas of interest:

- Using call and response can have an aerobic benefit.

- For maximum aerobic benefit, reciting poetry should be combined with movement.

- The scientists were led to conduct the study because of therapists' observations that creative arts were helping their patients.

Combing through these studies, I believe that:

- Using the technique of call and response, combined with movement, causes synapses in the brain to fire in such a way that a person with memory loss retains the words of the poem long enough to repeat them.

- People with dementia can draw from echoic memory when poetry is recited to them, and repeating the lines of a poem causes brain synapses to fire and engages a person's brain and memory.

- By using rhyming and rhythmic poetry, the end rhymes function as almost a magnet to draw the brain to the rhyme word.

- Rhyme words may act as memory devises.

- Guiding a person living with dementia in a language activity causes increased synaptic activity in the brain that stimulates recall. What you see is the person laughing or smiling, and their affect brightened.

Other Studies and Writing on Poetry and Memory

The authors of a study entitled, "A Narrative Analysis of Poetry Written from the Words of People Given a Diagnosis of Dementia," found that, "there is significant emotional and psychological benefit gained from being able to access the creative part of one's identity." (http://dem.sagepub.com/content/early/2013/05/22/1471301213488116.abstract)

The study "Using Poetry to Improve the Quality of Life and Care for People with Dementia," found that, "reminiscence-based poetry activities can improve the quality of life and care for persons with dementia, helping to restore their 'personhood' in the eyes of those who care for them." (http://www.tandfonline.com/doi/abs/10.1080/17533015.2011.584885#preview)

In 2009, the APP was the subject of a research project, "Observation of Behaviors Among Memory-Impaired Adults During a Poetry Reading," which the author, Lynn Green, wrote for her Master of Science in Nursing from Indiana Wesleyan University. (http://www.alzpoetry.com/Research/) Green's describes the study and her observations:

> Poetry provided the conduit for eight memory-impaired participants to express their memories in a caring environment. From the observations, poetry emerged as a positive intervention that allows for human connection and the resurfacing of self.

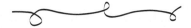

The following are a few thoughts on the background research I have done on the "biology of poetry":

- Poetry was first used as a way to record the stories of our communities.

- Our brains and neural networks were formed such that rhyme and rhythm were central to us as humans and worked as memory devises.

- Reciting poetry, especially when combined with movement, has an aerobic benefit by increasing oxygen flow to the brain.

- Unusual and beautiful use of language stimulates the language center of the brain.

- Seeing people living with dementia perform and create poetry may change the perceptions of their family members and caregivers; the person with dementia is viewed with more compassion and is seen more as someone who still has the ability to be engaged and less through the lens of the disease.

As we are seeing similar findings in art, dance, music, story-telling, and theater, it is my belief that nonpharmacological approaches will take the lead in providing a better quality of life and more humane care for people living with memory loss and their family members.

Step B: List Materials

The following materials will be used in our investigation:

- Four poems grouped around a theme:
  - ~ "The Tyger," by William Blake
  - ~ "The Purple Cow," by Gelett Burgess
  - ~ "The Eagle," by Alfred Lord Tennyson
  - ~ "The Raven" (opening stanza), by Edgar Allan Poe

- One poetry session leader

- One scribe

- Ten people with a diagnosis of Alzheimer's disease or related dementia

- Five observers for a live session and five observers to observe the video recording of the session

- Two video cameras

Step C: List Steps

We will observe and describe the behaviors of 10 individuals with memory impairment during 8, 1-hour poetry sessions held once a week for 2 months. We will record their behaviors on video for use to further observe and describe their behaviors. We will train the observers in looking for and describing:

- Positive facial expressions

- Verbal engagement

- Positive emotional reactions

- Negative emotional reactions

Each observer will be assigned two people and will track their responses by writing a description at a minimum of ever 4 minutes for each person. The observers using the video recorders will follow a similar process of observation, but will have the ability to stop the recording to allow more time to write their observations.

Step D: Estimate Time

We will observe and describe the behaviors of the group once a week for 2 months during a period of 1 hour during which they are not engaged in an art activity. The observers will follow the same procedure of observation.

Step E: Analyze and Communicate

We will analyze our data, draw a conclusion, and communicate our results. Our goal is for this initial research to lead to further studies of dementia arts on a national basis.

Conclusion

As a life-time student of poetry, I find it fascinating to explore how poetry might relate to brain science. Moreover, over the past 10 years conducting hundreds of poetry sessions for people living with memory loss, I see poetry work on a daily basis in the smiles, laughter, and warmth of the people I have had the honor to serve.

While the studies sited in this section are of small samples of participants, they are pointing to hard evidence of the effectiveness of poetry. And we believe our own research, first with Lynn Green and now embarking on working with the Dementia Arts Research Ensemble, will show strong evidence that poetry and other arts provide a rich stimulus to improve the quality of life of people living with Alzheimer's disease and related dementia.

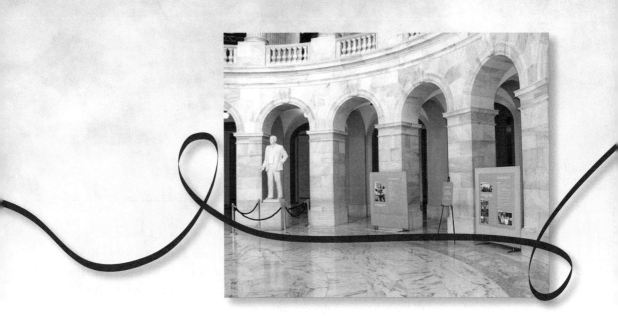

Epilogue
The Senator's Ear

At the Alzheimer's Foundation of America conference in Washington, D.C., in March of 2012, we were encouraged to visit our U.S. representatives and ask them to support the National Alzheimer's Project Plan (NAPA) (Public Law 111-375), which Congress passed unanimously in December 2010 and was signed into law by President Barack Obama in January 2011. NAPA requires the creation of a national strategic plan to address the rapidly escalating Alzheimer's disease crisis and the coordination of Alzheimer's disease efforts across the federal government. This is the first time that the United States has had a national response to Alzheimer's disease and related dementia.

As I have homes in both New Mexico and New York, I decided to try and meet with New Mexico Senator Tom Udall's staff. I was happy when they invited me to have coffee with other New Mexicans visiting D.C. that week and even happier to learn that Senator Udall would be hosting the occasion.

When I arrived, his staff ushered me into the waiting room of his office. A staffer then announced that we could take a photograph with the senator. As he put his arm around me to pose for the photo, I said to him, "I do poetry with people living with Alzheimer's disease, and in New Mexico we work a lot in Spanish. Would you like to hear one of the little Spanish poems, or *dichos*, we use?" Senator Udall stepped back, took a look at me, and said that he would like to hear one. I recited the following to him:

Pan es pan, queso es queso
no hay amor sino hay un beso.

The Senator did not need the English translation and started laughing.

Bread is bread, cheese is cheese
There is no love, unless you kiss me.

He said to his staff, "Make sure you write down that *dicho* that Gary shared with me. I want to remember that."

At the coffee get together I met other constituents from New Mexico, including a group of hotshot firefighters, soldiers from the National Guard, and rocket scientists from Los Alamos. Everyone was friendly and chatting, and the Senator's staff circulated making sure everyone was comfortable.

Senator Udall entered and gave a talk acknowledging all of the groups that were represented in the room by saying a little about each one and how our good work helped make New Mexico a better place to live. When he got to me, he told the group about the *dicho* I had shared with him and if I would like to recite it. I said the *dicho* and as I got to the part about kissing, I repeated "beso . . . beso . . . beso" in a kind of chant and then through my arms open and shouted, "abrazo," or "hug" in Spanish. As I shouted, I lunged for the biggest National Guard soldier, who was over 6 feet tall and wearing a big black cowboy hat, which made him seem even taller. He hugged me back and said, "I'm sure glad you didn't kiss me."

The room broke out in laughter. Every chance I get I hope to introduce poetry in a way that will change people's minds about how useful and funny it can be. There in the Senator's office I wanted the group to feel that in that moment poetry brought them together, that even if they felt they do not like or perhaps even hate poetry, a poem gave them a belly laugh.

Later the solider pulled me aside and said quietly, "I don't want the other guys to hear this, but when I was a little boy my grandmother used to sing me to sleep with a *dicho*. You brought back those memories to me today and made me cry a little." Then he softly sang the *dicho*.

After coffee I met with Jeanette Lukens, the Senior Legislative Assistant for Senator Udall. The rule of thumb is you are supposed to give your talk in 5 minutes, to state your case quickly (otherwise you are taking up too much of their time). Instead, Jeanette and I spoke for almost an hour, laughing and talking about poetry and New Mexico.

Later that day, back at the Alzheimer's Foundation of America conference, Mary Alice Parker, a staffer for then Congressman and now Senator Edward Markey, the lead author of NAPA, spoke to the conference attendees about the plan. When her talk was over, I introduced myself. When I told her I write poetry with people living with Alzheimer's disease, she said, "We should have an art show on Capitol Hill." I told her about meeting with Jeanette and that I was sure Senator Udall would support the project.

I met with Mary Alice and Jeanette a few weeks later, and the art show project was born.

Dementia Arts on Capitol Hill

Whispering into the Senator's ear led directly to the creation of Dementia Arts on Capitol Hill (DACH). The project's mission was to give the creativity of people navigating memory loss a national showcase and bring to the forefront this powerful response to America's aging population, as well as to provide compelling examples to answer the question of what can be done today to improve the quality of life of people living with dementia and their families.

DACH was co-produced by the Alzheimer's Poetry Project and the National Center for Creative Aging, and partner organizations include the Alzheimer's Association, Washington, D.C., chapter; the Center on Aging, Heath, and Humanities; Generations United; Iona Senior Services; and Society for Arts and Healthcare

Highlights of DACH include the following:

- More than 5,000 people passed through the Rotunda of the Russell Senate Office Building during the exhibit from September 17 to September 21, 2012.

- More than 300 people attended 7 outreach arts events as part of the Dementia Arts Festival at Washington, D.C., assisted living and adult day centers. More than 15 new works of art, including dances, poems, and songs, were created for the project.

- More than 100 people attended the culminating event and reception at the Memory Arts Café at Iona Senior Services.

- The research panel briefing was standing room only, with more than 100 people in attendance. Senator Tom Udall and Rocco Landesman, Chairman of the National Endowment of the Arts, spoke at the event.

- Testimony at the research panel briefing included preliminary research that showed quality of life is improved and healthcare cost savings may be attained through the use of arts programming for people living with dementia.

You may read more about Dementia Arts on Capitol Hill at http://dementiaarts.com/.

Dementia Arts Research Ensemble

One of the results of organizing DACH was the formation of the Dementia Arts Research Ensemble (DARE). Working in partnership with the National Center for Creative Aging, the Alzheimer's Poetry Project, KAIROS Alive!, Meet Me at MoMA, Songwriting Works™, and TimeSlips, a research coalition was formed in partnership with Kate de Medeiros, Ph.D., Assistant Professor of Gerontology and Scripps Fellow, Miami University; Jennifer M. Kinney, Ph.D., Professor, Department of Sociology & Gerontology, Scripps Research Fellow, and Affiliate, Department of Psychology; and Daniel Kaplan, Ph.D., Columbia University School of Social Work and postdoctoral research fellow at the Institute for Geriatric Psychiatry at Weill Cornell Medical College. In an excerpt from our first research proposal written for the National Institute of Health, Dr. de Medeiros notes:

> One of the primary goals of dementia research has been to find successful interventions that slow disease progress and/or restore lost abilities. Increasingly, dementia care interventions that utilize the cultural arts (e.g., dance, storytelling, music) have gained attention for their ability to generate significant social and behavioral changes, although enthusiasm for their success has been dampened by methodological weakness (e.g., small sample sizes, lack of randomized design).

> To better understand how the cultural arts effect change, several things are needed: a basic understanding of how the cultural arts operate, the mechanisms that are involved, what behavioral and emotional benefits are present, at what level change occurs (e.g., individual, larger cultural units), and how often benefits should be measured.

It is an honor to work with my colleagues in forming DARE and in pushing forward our ability to improve the lives of people living with dementia.

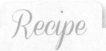

LUCKY BABY LULLABY

INGREDIENTS:

1 soldier
1 poet

INSTRUCTIONS:

Mix love of words with love of family. Stir in grandma or abuela's voice. She is singing my son, or mijo. You fall asleep to her song, or dicho. Years later you remember this moment and share it with a stranger to help him on his way.

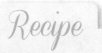
Recipe

ART AND GERONTOLOGY STEW

INGREDIENTS:

artists
dancers
musicians
poets
storytellers
scientists

INSTRUCTIONS:

Stir gently, until frothy.

This may be the most important lesson in being creative. Don't be afraid to reach out to people and ask for help. Ask to collaborate. Offer to help. For many of you who are caring for a loved one, you will need help, and on the flip side it feels great to offer help. For people who are professional caregivers, call the local school and talk to the drama teacher or call the ballet and ask for dancers to come to your facility.

By asking for the scientists to help, we are on the path to do research and to identify what is happening in a dementia arts session. That moment of shear joy when a person with memory loss seemingly wakes up, smiles, laughs, and becomes more social. That powerful moment of creativity and play we all want in our days.

What will your stew be made of? Please do not feel as though you must do this alone. We want to hear from you. Feel free to please reach out, we are here to help (Gary@alzpoetry.com).

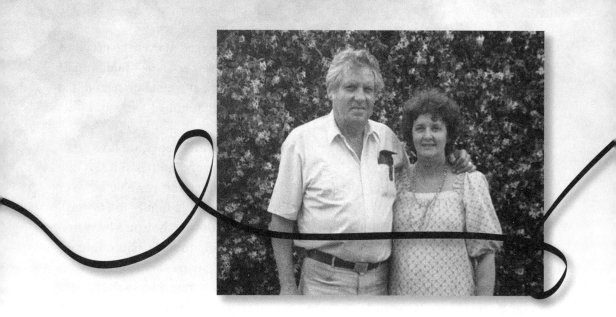

Coda

The coda in Italian is the tail, and in music it brings a piece to an end. Let us go back to where my journey started with being a caregiver for my mother.

It was her flower shop. She had been working at the shop for a neighbor and when he wanted to sell it, she jumped at the chance to buy it from him. But she needed help. The first thing she needed was my father's support, and he gave it to her completely.

My father was retiring from his career at the U.S. Immigration and Naturalization Service. He had started as a Border Patrol Agent in a little town in Texas and rose in the ranks to be the Assistant District Director of Investigations, overseeing 300 field agents in the western United States.

He often talked of how that shift of responsibility from working at that level in law enforcement to being yelled at by a customer whose roses wilted prematurely affected him, but he jumped in and together he and my mother worked hard to build the flower business.

They also needed cash for the purchase, and so my grandfather, Louise Todd, made a loan to them. My father never got over how that loan, at the height of the recession in the early 1980s, had an extremely high interest rate and how much delight my rich farmer Papa took in that rate. When my parents sold the store to Margaret and me, they took pride in giving us a fair deal.

The one thing my mother did not need help with was studying and working hard at developing her skills as a flower designer. She grew and learned. She had a devoted following for her work, especially for her annual

Christmas show with holiday designs, which she worked at over the previous year. She always started planning for the next year as soon as the materials went on sale after Christmas; that way she got them at a good price and had all year to plan for her big show. I can still smell the mulled wine and pine boughs.

As my wife Margaret and I paid the loan off over 7 years, we loved that it helped my parents to travel and enjoy the end of my mother's life. While she enjoyed her freedom (they bought a motor home and traveled all over America, took trips abroad, and once brought the whole family to Hawaii), nothing made her happier than coming back to the flower shop on a busy holiday to help with centerpieces or at prom time to help to make boutonnieres.

Once, right after being diagnosed with cancer, my mother came to work and when I tried to tell her she should go home and rest, she looked at me and said, "I really want to be here." She stayed and worked along side us, happy with her flowers and creativity, and joking and gossiping with the staff.

Another time, when somehow I had misplaced the order for a bride's wedding flowers and was in a panic to make the bouquets and get them to the church on time, she rushed to the store, put on her apron, and said, "Where do we start? Don't worry, we can do this." That morning as we worked furiously she would look at me, laugh, and say "You are so lucky you have a nice mother." We made it with minutes to spare.

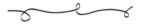

I am a lucky guy. I get to follow my dream of being a poet, to have poetry central to my life, to use poetry every day, to have people invite me into their home to share poetry with them, to use poetry with people at the end of their life, to be close to them.

When I recite a poem by Shakespeare, I am using the exact shape of his body; my synapses fire as his synapses fired, my brain lights up as his brain lit up, my lungs make the shape of his lungs to hold the air the poem rides on, my throat makes the shape his throat made, my tongue, my lips, my vocal cords all function just as his did and, in a sense, Shakespeare is back in the room with us. As you, too, say the poems, in a sense Shakespeare is inside you as well. These old poets want to be of use, they want their words to live, to be our lucky charms and give us insight into life.

To have found this wonderful way of using poetry to serve people who are living with memory loss or reaching the end of their life is such a gift. It has been such a pleasure to be with you. Thank you, for listening to my tale.

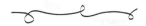

The Bird Feeder

"It's pretty bad when your life
gets down to watching birds," she says.

Here, let me open a field guide
and identify myself.

A yellow oriole flies in,
lifts the sheet and swaddles you.

Red hummingbirds swoop
into your gape,
you begin to flutter.

We wrap you
in a crescent
of crow feathers
and rattle songs
to your tumors.

Crimson cardinal
wings sprout
from your ankles.

You soar aloft.
A nest of thorns
falls from the sky.

You are flying
softly.

I press my ear
to your wend
and whirl,
to learn
your silence.

Resources

Advocacy Groups

Alzheimer's Foundation of America
http://www.alzfdn.org/

National Center for Creative Aging
http://www.creativeaging.org/

New York Memory Center
http://nymemorycenter.org/

Dementia Arts Groups

Art

Art and Minds
http://www.artsandminds.org/

Discover Your Story at the Minneapolis Institute of Arts http://new.artsmia.org/
visit/plan-your-trip/tours/

http://mia-wp-cdn.s3.amazonaws.com/wp-content/uploads/2013/06/DYS_Win-
ter_Spring13.pdf

Elders Share the Arts
http://www.estanyc.org/

GoldMind Arts and Aging
www.goldmindartsandaging.com

Meet Me at MoMA
http://www.moma.org/meetme/

Opening Minds through Art (OMA)
http://www.scrippsoma.org/

SPARK! Cultural Programming for People with Memory Loss
http://www.alz.org/sewi/in_my_community_19695.asp

Sweet Readers
http://www.sweetreaders.org/

The Creative Center at University Settlement
http://www.thecreativecenter.org/tcc/

Dance

BodyWise Dance
http://www.bodywisedance.com/

KAIROS Dancing Heart™
http://www.kairosdance.org/

Rhythm Break Cares
http://rhythmbreakcares.wordpress.com/

Music

Songwriting Works™
http://www.songwritingworks.org/

Storytelling

Story Core Memory Loss Initiative
http://storycorps.org/memory-loss/

Time*Slips*™
http://www.timeslips.org/

Theater

Stagebridge Senior Theatre
http://stagebridge.org/

Films

Alive Inside
www.BeAliveInside.com

*Five Pocket Films to Increase Understanding of
a 21st Century Epidemic: A Quick Look at Alzheimer's*
http://www.aboutalz.org/

I Remember Better When I Paint
http://www.irememberbetterwhenipaint.com/

The Genius of Marian
http://geniusofmarian.com/

Poetry

Alzheimer's Poetry Project
http://www.alzpoetry.com/

Dementia Positive
http://www.dementiapositive.co.uk/

Books

Alzheimer's from the Inside Out, by Richard Taylor (Health Professionals Press, 2007).

Beyond Forgetting: Poetry and Prose about Alzheimer's Disease, edited by Holly J. Hughes (The Kent State University Press, 2009).

Dear Alzheimer's: A Caregiver's Diary & Poems, by Esther Altshul Helgott (Cave Moon Press, 2013).

Forget Memory: Creating Better Lives for People with Dementia, by Anne Davis Basting, (The Johns Hopkins University Press, 2009).

I Never Told Anybody: Teaching Poetry Writing to Old People, by Kenneth Koch (Teachers and Writers Collaborative, 1997).

In Search of Memory: The Emergence of a New Science of Mind, by Eric Kandel (W. W. Norton & Company, 2007).

MeetMe: Making Art Accessible to People with Dementia, by Francesca Rosenberg, Amir Parsa, Laurel Humble, and Carrie McGee (The Museum of Modern Art, 2009).

Musicophilia: Tales of Music and the Brain, by Oliver Sacks (Vintage Books, 2007).

Nine Gates: Entering the Mind of Poetry, by Jane Hirshfield (HarperPerennial, 1997).

The MIX@GES Experience: How to Promote Intergenerational Bonding Through Creative Digital Media, by Almuth Fricke, Maureen Marley, Alice Morton, and Julia Thomé (European Grundvig, 2013).

The Age of Insight: The Quest to Understand the Unconscious in Art, Mind, and Brain, From Vienna 1900 to the Present, by Eric R. Kandel (Random House, 2012).

The Forgetting: Alzheimer's: Portrait of an Epidemic, by David Shenk (Doubleday, 2001; reprint edition Anchor, 2003).

The Long Hello: The Other Side of Alzheimer's, by Cathy Borrie (Nightwing Press, 2010).

The Alzheimer's Project: Momentum in Science, by John Hoffman and Susan Fromke (HBO, 2009).

What Are Old People For? How Elders Will Save the World, by William H. Thomas, M.D. (VanderWyk & Brunham, 2007).

First Lines of Poems